Evidence-based Clinical Chinese Medicine

Volume 20
Chronic Cough

Evidence-based Clinical Chinese Medicine

Print ISSN: 2529-7562
Online ISSN: 2529-7554

Series Co Editors-in-Chief

Charlie Changli Xue *(RMIT University, Australia)*
Chuanjian Lu *(Guangdong Provincial Hospital of Chinese Medicine, China)*

Published

More information on this series can also be found at https://www.worldscientific.com/series/ebccm

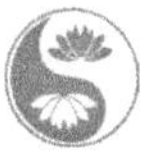

Evidence-based Clinical Chinese Medicine

Co Editors-in-Chief

Charlie Changli Xue
RMIT University, Australia

Chuanjian Lu
Guangdong Provincial Hospital of Chinese Medicine, China

Volume 20
Chronic Cough

Lead Authors

Johannah Shergis
RMIT University, Australia

Yuanbin Chen
Guangdong Provincial Hospital of Chinese Medicine, China

World Scientific

NEW JERSEY · LONDON · SINGAPORE · BEIJING · SHANGHAI · HONG KONG · TAIPEI · CHENNAI · TOKYO

Published by

World Scientific Publishing Co. Pte. Ltd.

5 Toh Tuck Link, Singapore 596224

USA office: 27 Warren Street, Suite 401-402, Hackensack, NJ 07601

UK office: 57 Shelton Street, Covent Garden, London WC2H 9HE

Library of Congress Cataloging-in-Publication Data
Names: Xue, Charlie Changli, author. | Lu, Chuan-jian, 1964–   author.
Title: Evidence-based clinical Chinese medicine / Charlie Changli Xue, Chuanjian Lu.
Description: New Jersey : World Scientific, 2016. | Includes bibliographical references and index.
Identifiers: LCCN 2015030389| ISBN 9789814723084 (v. 1 : hardcover : alk. paper) |
    ISBN 9789814723091 (v. 1 : paperback : alk. paper) |
    ISBN 9789814723121 (v. 2 : hardcover : alk. paper) |
    ISBN 9789814723138 (v. 2 : paperback : alk. paper) |
    ISBN 9789814759045 (v. 3 : hardcover : alk. paper) |
    ISBN 9789814759052 (v. 3 : paperback : alk. paper)
Subjects: | MESH: Medicine, Chinese Traditional--methods. | Clinical Medicine--methods. |
    Evidence-Based Medicine--methods. | Psoriasis. | Pulmonary Disease, Chronic Obstructive.
Classification: LCC RC81 | NLM WB 55.C4 | DDC 616--dc23
LC record available at http://lccn.loc.gov/2015030389

Volume 20: Chronic Cough
ISBN 978-981-122-313-6 (hardcover)
ISBN 978-981-123-543-6 (paperback)
ISBN 978-981-122-314-3 (ebook for institutions)
ISBN 978-981-122-315-0 (ebook for individuals)

British Library Cataloguing-in-Publication Data
A catalogue record for this book is available from the British Library.

For any available supplementary material, please visit
https://www.worldscientific.com/worldscibooks/10.1142/11906#t=suppl

Disclaimer

The information in this book is based on systematic analyses of the best available evidence for Chinese medicine interventions both historical and contemporary. Every effort has been made to ensure accuracy and completeness of the data herein. This book is intended for clinicians, researchers and educators. The practice of evidence-based medicine consists of consideration of the best available evidence, practitioners' clinical experience and judgment, and patients' preference. Not all interventions are acceptable in all countries. It is important to note that some of the substances mentioned in this book may no longer be in use, may be toxic, or may be prohibited or restricted under the provisions of the Convention on International Trade in Endangered Species of Wild Fauna and Flora (CITES). Practitioners, researchers and educators are advised to comply with the relevant regulations in their country and with the restrictions on the trade in species included in CITES appendices I, II and III. This book is not intended as a guide for self-medication. Patients should seek professional advice from qualified Chinese medicine practitioners.

Foreword

Since the late 20th century, Chinese medicine, including acupuncture and herbal medicine, has been increasingly used throughout the world. The parallel development and spread of evidence-based medicine has provided challenges and opportunities for Chinese medicine. The opportunities have been evidence-based medicine's emphasis on the effective use of the best available clinical evidence, incorporating the clinicians' clinical experience, subject to patients' preference. Such practices have a patient focus which reflects the historical nature of Chinese medicine practice. However, the challenges are also significant due to the fact that, despite the long-term development and very rich literature accumulated over 2,000 years, there is an overall lack of high-level clinical evidence for many of the interventions used in Chinese medicine.

To address this knowledge gap, we need to generate clinical evidence through high-quality clinical studies and to evaluate evidence to enable effective use of such available evidence to promote evidence-based Chinese medicine practice.

Modern Chinese medicine is rooted in its classical literature and the legacies of ancient doctors, grounded in the practice of expert clinicians and increasingly informed by clinical and experimental research efforts. In recognition of the unique features of Chinese medicine, for each of the conditions in this series a 'whole-evidence' approach is used to provide a synthesis of different types and levels of evidence to enable practitioners to make clinical decisions informed by the current best evidence.

There are four main components of this 'whole-evidence' approach. In the first component, we present the current approaches to the diagnosis, differentiation and treatment of each condition based on expert consensus in published textbooks and clinical guidelines. This provides an overview of how the condition is currently managed. The second component provides an analysis of the condition in historical context based on systematic searches of the *Zhong Hua Yi Dian* which includes the full texts of more than 1,000 classical medical books. These analyses provide objective views on how the condition has been treated over two millennia, reveal continuities and discontinuities between traditional and modern practice, and suggest avenues for future research.

The third component is the assessment of evidence derived from modern clinical studies of Chinese medicine interventions. The methods established by the *Cochrane Collaboration* are used as the basis for conducting systematic reviews and undertaking meta-analyses of outcome data for randomised controlled trials (RCTs). In addition, the clinical relevance of meta-analysis data is enhanced by examining the herbal formulas, individual herbs and acupuncture treatments that were assessed in the RCTs and the evidence base is broadened by the inclusion of data from controlled clinical trials and non-controlled studies. The fourth component is to determine how the herbal medicine interventions may achieve the effects indicated by the clinical trials. Thus for each of the most frequently used herbs we provide reviews of their effects in pre-clinical models and their likely mechanisms of action.

For each condition, this 'whole-evidence' approach links clinical expertise, historical precedent, clinical research data and experimental research to provide the reader with assessments of the current state of the evidence for the efficacy, effectiveness and safety of Chinese medicine interventions using herbal medicines, acupuncture and moxibustion, and other health care practices such as *tai chi*.

Since these books are available in Chinese and English, they can benefit patients, practitioners and educators internationally and enable practitioners to make clinical decisions informed by the current best evidence.

These publications represent a major milestone in the development of Chinese medicine and make a significant contribution to the development of evidence-based Chinese medicine globally.

Co-editors-in-Chief

Distinguished Professor Charlie Changli Xue,
RMIT University, Australia

Professor Chuanjian Lu, Guangdong Provincial Hospital of
Chinese Medicine, China

Purpose of This Book

This book is intended for clinicians, researchers and educators. It can be used to inform tertiary education and clinical practice by providing systematic, multidimensional assessments of the best available evidence for using Chinese medicine to manage each common clinical condition.

How to Use This Book

Some Definitions

A glossary is included, containing terms and definitions which frequently appear in the book. It also describes the definitions of statistical tests, methodological terms, evaluation tools and interventions. For example, in this book, integrative medicine refers to the combined use of a Chinese medicine treatment with conventional medical management, and combination therapies refer to two or more Chinese medicines from different therapy groups (e.g. Chinese herbal medicine, acupuncture or other Chinese medicine therapies) administered together. Terminology used throughout the book is based on the World Health Organisation's *Standard Terminologies on Traditional Medicine in the Western Pacific Region* (2007) where possible or from the cited reference.

Data Analysis and Interpretation of Results

In order to synthesise the clinical evidence, a range of statistical analysis approaches are used. In general, the effect size for dichotomous data is reported as a risk ratio (RR) with 95% confidence intervals (CI), and for continuous data, they are reported as mean difference (MD) with 95% CI. Statistically significant effects are indicated with an asterisk*. Readers should note that statistical significance does not necessarily correspond with a clinically important effect. Interpretation of results should take into consideration the clinical significance, quality of studies (expressed as high, low or unclear risk of bias in this book) and heterogeneity amongst the studies. Tests for heterogeneity are conducted using the I^2 statistic. An I^2 score greater than 50% may indicate substantial heterogeneity.

Use of Evidence in Practice

The Grading of Recommendations Assessment, Development and Evaluation (GRADE) approach was used to summarise the results and certainty of the evidence for critical and important comparisons and outcomes. Due to the diverse nature of Chinese medicine practice, treatment recommendations are not included with the summary of findings tables. Therefore, readers will need to interpret the evidence with reference to the local practice environment.

Limitations

Readers should note some of the methodological limitations of the classical literature and the clinical evidence.

- Search terms used to search the *Zhong Hua Yi Dian* database may not include all terms that have been used for the condition, which may alter the findings.
- Chinese language has changed over time. Citations have been interpreted for analysis, and such interpretations may be subject to disagreement.
- Chinese medicine theory has evolved over time. As such, concepts described in classical Chinese medical literature may no longer be found in contemporary works.
- Symptoms described in citations may be common to many conditions, and a judgment was required to determine the likelihood of

the citation being related to the condition. This may have introduced some bias due to the subjective nature of the judgment.

- The vast majority of the clinical evidence for Chinese medicine treatments has come from China. The applicability of the findings to other populations and other countries requires further assessment.
- Many studies included participants with varying disease severity. Where possible, subgroup analyses were undertaken to examine the effects in different subpopulations. As this was not always possible, the findings may be limited to the population included, and not to subpopulations.
- The potential risk of bias found in many included studies suggested methodological limitations. The findings for GRADE assessments based on studies of very low- to moderate-quality evidence should be interpreted accordingly.
- Nine major English- and Chinese-language databases were searched to identify clinical studies, in addition to clinical trial registers. Other studies may exist which were not identified through searches, and which may alter the findings.
- The calculation of frequency of herbal formula use was based on formula names. It is possible that studies evaluated herbal treatments with the same or similar herb ingredients, but which were given different formula names. Due to the complexity of herbal formulas, it was considered not appropriate to make a judgment as to the similarity of formulas for analysis. As such, the frequency of formulas reported in Chapter 5 may be underestimated.
- The most frequently utilised herbs which may have contributed to the treatment effect have been described in Chapter 5. These herbs may provide leads for further exploration. Calculation of the herbs with potential effect is based on frequency of formulas reported in the studies, and does not take into consideration the clinical implications and functions of every herb in a formula.

Authors and Contributors

Co-editors-in-Chief
Distinguished Prof. Charlie Changli Xue (*RMIT University, Australia*)
Prof. Chuanjian Lu (*Guangdong Provincial Hospital of Chinese Medicine, China*)

Co-Deputy Editors-in-Chief
Assoc. Prof. Anthony Lin Zhang (*RMIT University, Australia*)
Dr. Brian H May (*RMIT University, Australia*)
Prof. Xinfeng Guo (*Guangdong Provincial Hospital of Chinese Medicine, China*)
Prof. Zehuai Wen (*Guangdong Provincial Hospital of Chinese Medicine, China*)

Lead Authors
Dr. Johannah Shergis (*RMIT University, Australia*)
Dr. Yuanbin Chen (*Guangdong Provincial Hospital of Chinese Medicine, China*)

Co-authors
RMIT University (Australia):
Assoc. Prof. Anthony Lin Zhang
Distinguished Prof. Charlie Changli Xue
Guangdong Provincial Hospital of Chinese Medicine (China):

Prof. Lin Lin
Prof. Lei Wu
Prof. Xinfeng Guo
Dr. Zhenhu Wu
Dr. Han Xie
Prof. Chuanjian Lu

Members of Advisory Committee and Panel

CO-CHAIRS OF PROJECT PLANNING COMMITTEE
Prof. Peter J Coloe (*RMIT University, Australia*)
Prof. Yubo Lyu (*Guangdong Provincial Hospital of Chinese Medicine, China*)
Prof. Dacan Chen (*Guangdong Provincial Hospital of Chinese Medicine, China*)

CENTRE ADVISORY COMMITTEE (IN ALPHABETICAL ORDER)
Prof. Keji Chen (*The Chinese Academy of Sciences, China*)
Prof. Aiping Lu (*Hong Kong Baptist University, China*)
Prof. Caroline Smith (*University of Western Sydney, Australia*)
Prof. David F Story (*RMIT University, Australia*)

METHODOLOGY EXPERT ADVISORY PANEL (IN ALPHABETICAL ORDER)
Prof. Zhaoxiang Bian (*Hong Kong Baptist University, China*)
The Late Prof. George Lewith (*University of Southampton, United Kingdom*)
Prof. Lixing Lao (*The University of Hong Kong, China*)
Prof. Jianping Liu (*Beijing University of Chinese Medicine, China*)
Prof. Frank Thien (*Monash University, Australia*)
Prof. Jialiang Wang (*Sichuan University, China*)

CONTENT EXPERT ADVISORY PANEL (IN ALPHABETICAL ORDER)
Prof. Frank Thien (*Monash University, Australia*)
Dr. Christopher Worsnop (*Austin Health, Australia*)
Prof. Kefang Lai (*The First Affiliated Hospital of Guangzhou Medical University, China*)
Prof. Jia Zhu (*Jiangsu Provincial Hospital of Chinese Medicine, China*)

Distinguished Professor Charlie Changli Xue

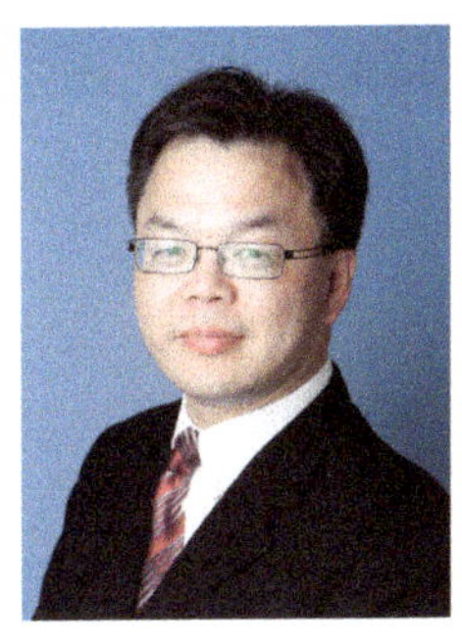

Distinguished Professor Charlie Changli Xue holds a Bachelor of Medicine (majoring in Chinese Medicine) from Guangzhou University of Chinese Medicine, China (1987) and a PhD from RMIT University, Australia (2000). He has been an academic, researcher, regulator and practitioner for almost three decades. Professor Xue has made significant contributions to evidence-based educational development, clinical research, regulatory framework and policy development, and provision of high-quality clinical care to the community. Professor Xue is recognised internationally as an expert in evidence-based traditional medicine and integrative health care.

Professor Xue is the Inaugural National Chair of the Chinese Medicine Board of Australia appointed by the Australian Health Workforce Ministerial Council (in 2011), and he was reappointed for a second term in 2014. Since 2007, he has been a Member of the World Health Organisation (WHO) Expert Advisory Panel for Traditional and Complementary Medicine, Geneva. Professor Xue is also Honorary Senior Principal Research Fellow at the Guangdong Provincial Academy of Chinese Medical Sciences, China.

At RMIT, Professor Xue is Executive Dean, School of Health and Biomedical Sciences. He is also Director, WHO Collaborating Centre for Traditional Medicine.

Between 1995 and 2010, Professor Xue was Discipline Head of Chinese Medicine at RMIT University. He leads the development of five successful undergraduate and postgraduate degree programmes in Chinese Medicine at RMIT University which is now a global leader in Chinese medicine education and research.

Professor Xue's research has been supported by research grants of over AUD15 million, including six project grants from the Australian Government's National Health and Medical Research Council (NHMRC) and two Australian Research Council (ARC) grants. He has contributed over 200 publications and has been frequently invited as keynote speaker for numerous national and international conferences. Professor Xue has contributed to over 300 media interviews on issues related to complementary medicine education, research, regulation and practice.

Professor Chuanjian Lu

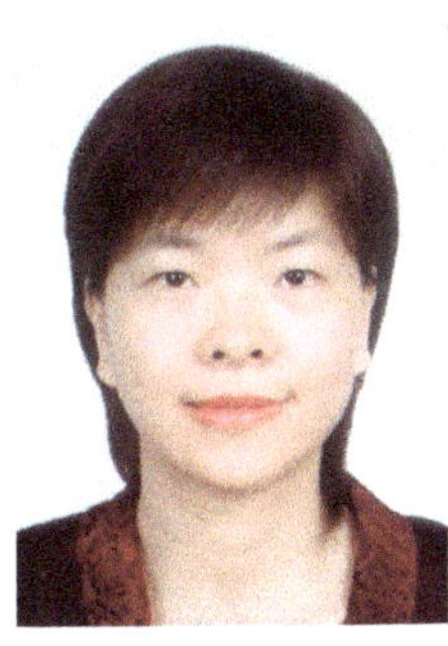

Professor Chuanjian Lu is the Vice-president of Guangdong Provincial Hospital of Chinese Medicine (Guangdong Provincial Academy of Chinese Medical Sciences, Second Clinical Medical College of Guangzhou University of Chinese Medicine). She also is the Chair of the Guangdong Traditional Chinese Medicine (TCM) Standardisation Technical Committee, and the Vice-chair of the Immunity Specialty Committee of the World Federation of Chinese Medicine Societies (WFCMS).

Professor Lu has engaged in scientific research into TCM, clinical practice and teaching for some 25 years. Her research has been devoted to integrating traditional and western medicine. She has edited and published 12 monographs and 120 academic research articles as first author and corresponding author with over 30 articles being included in SCI journals.

She has received widespread recognition for her achievements with awards for Excellent Teacher of South China, National Outstanding Women TCM Doctor and National Outstanding Young Doctor of TCM. She also received the Science and Technology Star of the Association of Chinese Medicine, the National Excellent Science and Technology Workers of China Award and the Five-continent Women's Scientific Awards of China Medical Women's Association.

Professor Lu has won the Award of Science and Technology Progress over ten times from Guangdong Provincial Government, China Association of Chinese Medicine and Chinese Hospital Association.

Acknowledgements

The authors and contributors would like to acknowledge the valuable contributions of the following people who assisted with database searches, data extraction, data screening, data assessment, translation of documents, editing, and/or administrative tasks: Kevin Wang, Dr. Jhodie Duncan, Anje Scarfe, Feiting Fan, Yun Cai, Jianya Yang and Zehui Lin.

Contents

Contents

List of Figures

List of Tables

1

Introduction to Chronic Cough

OVERVIEW

Coughing is an important mechanism to clear the throat and lungs. However, in some people it can become bothersome and chronic, and is one of the most common reasons for people to seek medical attention. Chronic cough is defined as a cough for at least eight weeks, impacting about 10% of the adult population worldwide. There are many causes of chronic cough but the most common are asthma, rhinitis and reflux.

Definition of Chronic Cough

Coughing is an essential reflex that clears the larynx, trachea and bronchi of mucus secretions, noxious substances and foreign particles.[1] It involves a complicated pathophysiology of inspiration and expiration. Cough is the most common reason for patients to seek medical attention and often presents after an upper respiratory tract infection.[2,3] In most cases it is self-limiting, lasting a few days to a few weeks. However, if the cough lasts for more than eight weeks, it is classified as chronic cough[4-6] which is associated with significant morbidity and impairment to quality of life.[5-8] Chronic cough can be caused by several underlying conditions including cough variant asthma (CVA), upper airway cough syndrome (UACS), gastro-oesophageal reflux disease (GORD), infections (bronchitis, pneumonia, tuberculosis), eosinophilic bronchitis, chronic obstructive pulmonary disease (COPD), pulmonary fibrosis, bronchiectasis, interstitial lung disease, cancer, environmental exposures to dust or chemicals, or medications such as angiotensin-converting enzyme (ACE) inhibitors.[2]

Clinical Presentation and Subtypes of Chronic Cough

Due to a multitude of potential causes, differential diagnosis of chronic cough is important. Impact on health status and quality of life may also vary from trivial to severe. The three most common types of chronic cough, accounting for approximately 90% of cases, are CVA, UACS, and GORD.[9,10] In this book we have focused on these three types of chronic cough (Tables 1.1 and 1.2).

Cough Variant Asthma

Cough variant asthma is a form of asthma with bronchial hyper-responsiveness but without bronchospasm. It presents with dry, or minimally productive, cough especially at night, without the traditional asthma symptoms of wheezing and shortness of breath.[11] It was first described as 'variant asthma' in the early 1970s and later defined by Corrao *et al.* as CVA.[12,13] It is one of the most common causes of chronic cough and may have a worse prognosis than typical asthma.[2] Cough variant asthma presents with cough as the sole or predominant symptom, which is worse at night and often unproductive. It is considered to be a mild form of asthma because the typical airway narrowing observed in asthma (bronchoconstriction) is less severe

Table 1.1. Types of Chronic Cough Included in this Book

Type	Main Symptoms
Cough variant asthma (CVA)	Dry cough or minimally productive cough; worse at night
Upper airway cough syndrome (UACS)	Cough caused by mucus draining down the back of the throat; itchy and scratchy throat
Gastro-oesophageal reflux disease-related cough (GORD-C)	Cough, heartburn and acid reflux

and the symptoms are often reversible, with or without treatment. The severity of CVA ranges from mild to severe and intermittent to persistent. Mild symptoms cause few problems, but more severe CVA can impact quality of life and may be life-threatening. The cause is not clear but there are lifestyle and environmental factors that may increase the risk of developing CVA.[12,14]

Upper Airway Cough Syndrome

Upper airway cough syndrome, also known as postnasal drip syndrome, is the sensation of nasal secretions (or a drip) at the back of the throat. It is more recently referred to as UACS because it is unclear if the cough relates to postnasal drip, irritation or inflammation of the cough receptors. People with UACS have the urge to frequently clear their throat and may also have nasal congestion and discharge. Allergy evaluation, sinus imaging and nasopharyngoscopy may be useful to determine UACS but empirical treatment with antihistamines, decongestants or nasal corticosteroids may prove diagnostic.

Gastro-oesophageal Reflux Disease-related Cough

Gastro-oesophageal reflux disease-related cough (GORD-C) often goes unrecognised.[15,16] The cough is likely due to reflux causing increased sensitivity of the mucus membranes to gastric contents such as pepsin and inflammation in the larynx and pharynx. Symptoms of GORD typically include heartburn and regurgitation; however, it may also be asymptomatic. Not all patients with GORD-C will respond to acid suppression therapies or reflux treatment; however, trialling medication may assist with diagnosis.[5]

Epidemiology

Chronic cough is estimated to affect about 10% of people worldwide.[2,17] Populations in the Oceania region have the highest incidence (18.1%), followed by Europe (12.7%), North America (11%), South Asia (11.32%), China (11%) and Africa (2.3%).[17–20]

Chronic cough is more prevalent in the elderly and children, smokers and women.[21] Cough is the most common reason for consultation with a doctor[15] and estimates from the United States indicate that up to 38% of respiratory appointments are for chronic cough.[2] The sub-type of chronic cough may also vary by region; for example patients in the United States experience UACS more commonly than other types of chronic cough (UACS 41%, CVA 24% and GORD 21%),[22] compared to Asian countries such as China which report CVA 35.6%, UACS 18.6% and non-asthmatic eosinophilic bronchitis 17.2% as the most common types.[19]

Burden

Respiratory diseases are one of the largest contributors to the overall burden of disease globally.[23] The full extent of chronic cough burden for CVA, UACS and GORD-C is unknown as most population-based studies focus on COPD, asthma and infective respiratory diseases such as tuberculosis. Despite a paucity of research, it is still evident that the burden is significant. For example, asthma (CVA included) accounts for around 1% of all disability-adjusted life years (DALYs), approximately 16 million DALYs lost per year worldwide.[23] Health care costs contribute a large component of economic burden as people with chronic cough frequently seek out health care including recurrent doctor visits, hospitalisations, diagnostic tests and medications. This is evidenced in the United States where the annual cost of asthma is estimated at $81.9 billion.[24] Socio-economic burden including reduced activity days and hospital service utilisation is also substantial in Europe especially in asthmatics with chronic cough or phlegm.[25] Furthermore a considerable proportion of the disease burden (sometimes more than direct costs)[26] is caused by productivity loss and future earnings loss of people with chronic cough and their families.

Risk Factors

Females are more likely to develop chronic cough, possibly due to their heightened cough reflex sensitivity, especially in middle- to older-aged individuals.[6,27] Smokers are also at greater risk of developing chronic cough.[28] Other risk factors include obesity, rhinitis,[2,17] non-smokers with asthma or GORD, or ex-smokers with obesity.[28] Ethnic and genetic factors are less likely to play a role in chronic cough.

Environmental factors play a significant role in the development of chronic cough. For example, people in urban regions are at increased risk due to inhalation of irritants and pollutants. Occupational and environmental exposures can trigger chronic cough, and work-related exposures are estimated to affect 4–18% of people with cough.[29] In Beijing, China, people living close to major roads have a higher risk of chronic cough compared to other locations.[30] Indoor air pollution may also contribute to chronic cough in elderly populations.[31]

A number of factors can trigger CVA symptoms, and the triggers differ among individuals. Cough variant asthma risk factors include the typical asthma risk factors such as viral infections, exercise, exposure to allergens (house dust mites, pollens, mold spores and animals), environmental irritants (tobacco smoke, cold/dry air and fumes), foods (food chemicals/additives) and exercise. Cough variant asthma somewhat overlaps with allergic asthma, and people with CVA often have atopy and eczema or hay fever (allergic rhinitis), or food and drug allergies.[31] Seasonal variations in CVA are common and 40–80% of CVA suffers have atopy.[32]

Risk factors for other types of chronic cough can be used to differentiate CVA, UACS, and GORD. For example, ACE inhibitor medications can cause chronic cough in up to 5–35% of users.[33] The cough usually presents in the first few weeks of treatment but may also develop later. Once ACE inhibitors are stopped, the cough should recede within a few weeks. Viral airway infections can induce a persistent post-viral cough, possibly due to the airway sensory nerves being altered by the infection.

Pathological Processes

Coughing is a protective reflex that is triggered by chemical and mechanical stimuli. Cough receptors respond to stimuli and send signals through vagal afferent and superior laryngeal nerves to the cough centre and cerebral cortex. Muscles are then activated leading to cough. Chronic cough can cause airway inflammation and tissue remodelling leading to an ongoing enhanced cough reflex.[2] In people with chronic cough, there is distinct pathophysiology involving sensitisation of the cough reflex, such as neuronal hypersensitivity, increased activity of cough receptors, changes in the central response or brainstem sensitisation. This is coupled with higher cortical (voluntary) control of the cough reflex, indicating behavioural and psychological issues may play a part. Coupled together, these processes can lead to continued cough in the absence of the initiating stimuli.

People with CVA share similar pathophysiological features with typical asthma but the physiological abnormalities of CVA are more modest.[34] Cough variant asthma features include airway hyperresponsiveness, atopy and airway remodelling, as well as eosinophilic airway inflammation.[32] Mucosal biopsies have also shown structural changes including goblet cell hyperplasia, vascular proliferation and subepithelial thickening; therefore, anti-inflammatory treatment is recommended early in the management of CVA.[32] Inflammatory processes that may be involved in the cough mechanism include increased inflammatory mediators (e.g. histamine, prostaglandins and leukotrienes) and increased expression of capsaicin receptor TRPV-1, which is activated by a decrease in the pH of airway lining fluid.[32] Unlike asthma, people with CVA are likely to have normal lung function because airway narrowing is less obvious. Despite more modest physiological abnormalities, CVA patients can be difficult to treat because inhaled corticosteroid (ICS) treatments may have limited effectiveness.[35] This may be due to increased neutrophils in the airway mucosa leading to resistance to ICS treatment. Mast cells and goblet cell hyperplasia of bronchial epithelium appear to have less involvement in CVA compared to asthma.[36]

Upper airway cough syndrome is a syndrome, not a disease, therefore diagnosis can vary between patients. It can be caused by allergic and non-allergic rhinitis, chronic rhinosinusitis, infections or polyps. Research into the mechanisms underlying UACS has varied and a clear pathophysiology has not been determined. The most simplistic explanation is that nasal and sinus secretions drip into the pharynx and larynx, and stimulate cough receptors. More recently it was thought that UACS is caused by lower airway inflammation resulting from aspiration or mechanical stimulation from the cough itself. Inflammation is also thought to play a role, where inflammatory mediators stimulate cough receptors previously activated by a nervous reflex induced by inflammatory stimulation of nasal mucosa. Another theory is that there is increased cough sensitivity related to increased nasal neural activation and pharyngeal and/or laryngeal neural sensitivity.[37]

The mechanism of GORD-C is complex, and there are several potential mechanisms. When acid is introduced into the lower oesophagus, it precipitates a cough mediated by vagal nerves and there is a reflex between the lower oesophagus and the airways. Micro aspirations of contents such as acid and pepsin can also have a direct effect on the bronchial tree leading to bronchial hyper-responsiveness. Due to reflux, structural and inflammatory airway changes occur causing the repetitive coughing. Another theory is that reflux into the oesophagus causes mechanical and chemical stimulation of cough receptors.[15] Receptors in the muscles and submucosa may also be stimulated by muscle contraction in people with oesophageal dysmotility and spasm. Stimulation of oesophageal-bronchial interconnecting neural pathways may cause cough due to afferent nerve fibres of the vagus that run close to the trachea and oesophagus. There may also be positive feedback, whereby increased cough causes increased gastro-oesophageal reflux. In addition, GORD-C can be difficult to diagnose because some patients have limited, or no, gastrointestinal symptoms. However, these patients are often overweight and have high-calorie and fat diets.

Diagnosis

Chronic cough has many causes but there are some important features that distinguish the different types. The key diagnostic steps include initial evaluation of the symptoms, risk factors and aggravating factors. If the patient has a normal chest X-ray, is a non-smoker and is not receiving ACE inhibitors, CVA, UACS and GORD should be considered (Table 1.1).[5] The initial evaluation should include a detailed evaluation of symptoms, along with supplemental examinations such as lung function testing (spirometry), asthma challenge test, chest X-rays, cytological analysis of blood and phlegm, and 24-hour oesophageal pH monitoring to identify potential underlying conditions or warning symptoms (Fig. 1.1).

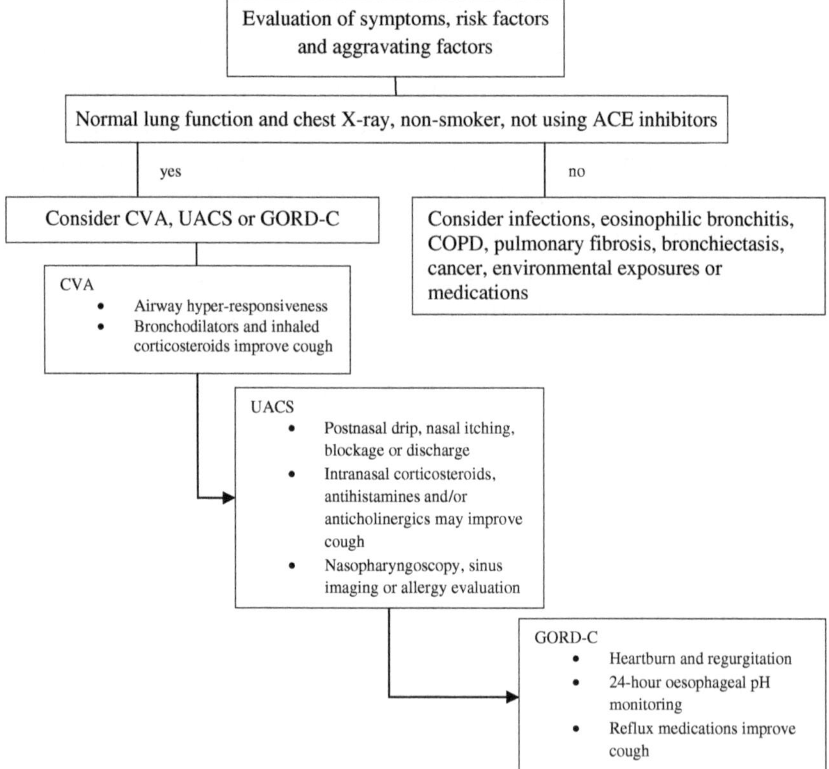

Fig. 1.1. Diagnostic flowchart of chronic cough.

Abbreviations: ACE, angiotensin-converting enzyme inhibitors; COPD, chronic obstructive pulmonary disease; CVA, cough variant asthma; GORD-C, gastro-oesophageal reflux disease-related cough; UACS, upper airway cough syndrome.

Some warnings may include smoking history, cough associated with voice abnormalities, hemoptysis, dyspnea, significant sputum production, hoarseness, fever, weight loss, hematemesis, dysphagia or recurrent pneumonia.[10,38] These symptoms may require further examination and may indicate a more serious cause of cough such as cancer.

All patients with chronic cough should undergo an asthma assessment.[5,10] Cough variant asthma presents as cough without wheezing and shortness of breath.[12] Differentiation can be achieved by examination and carefully noting down the patient's medical history. However, physical examination and pulmonary function may be normal. The key characteristics of CVA are airway hyper-responsiveness and improvement of cough after using bronchodilators such as beta-agonists. Responsiveness to bronchodilators or corticosteroids can be used as a diagnostic tool.[7] One of the main distinguishing features in asthma is airway sensitivity and hyper-responsiveness to triggers, especially a positive finding during challenge testing with products such as methacholine, whereas other causes of chronic cough, such as eosinophilic bronchitis, don't respond to the triggers.

Upper airway cough syndrome may be differentiated by the presence of symptoms indicative of nasal inflammation, such as postnasal drip, nasal itching, blockage, discharge or scratchy throat. Diagnosis of UACS is difficult because the chronic cough may be caused by many factors and attribution to one element, such as rhinitis, may be simplistic when, for example, asthma is also involved. A trial of UACS treatments, such as antihistamines and decongestants, may be initiated to help confirm the diagnosis before other diagnostic measures, such as imaging, nasopharyngoscopy or allergy evaluation, are undertaken.[5]

Gastro-oesophageal reflux disease should also be investigated in people with chronic cough. Typical GORD symptoms include heartburn and regurgitation, but some people may be asymptomatic and only present with chronic cough. The cough may become more apparent after meals or when talking but is less likely at night. Other symptoms may include the sensation of a lump or a tickle at the back of the throat, and a need to clear the throat. However, the presence or absence of cough in these situations is only suggestive of GORD, but not diagnostic. A thorough history is important because GORD is often misdiagnosed. The Reflux Cough Questionnaire can also be used to predict GORD-C when the score is greater than 20.[39] If GORD is suspected but testing is inconclusive, an empirical trial of anti-reflux medications may be a useful diagnostic alternative. To complicate diagnosis, some people may have more than one cause of cough; for example, any combination or permutation of CVA, UACS and GORD, or all three. Multimodality combination treatments may be necessary in these cases.

If treatment for the common causes is unsuccessful, other causes may be considered including non-asthmatic eosinophilic bronchitis. To rule out non-asthmatic eosinophilic bronchitis, a sputum sample should show less than 3% eosinophilic inflammation and patients usually respond to corticosteroid treatment. Furthermore, patients with non-asthmatic eosinophilic bronchitis can be differentiated due to no variable airflow obstruction and airway hyper-responsiveness.[40] Non-asthmatic pulmonary diseases should also be considered including COPD, bronchiolitis, interstitial lung disease, lung cancer, bronchiectasis, idiopathic pulmonary fibrosis and mycobacterial infection. Symptom assessment, a detailed history and lung function tests will help to differentiate other causes of chronic cough. Other causes may be cardiac arrhythmias or unknown refractory cough without an obvious medical aetiology.

Management

Chronic cough management is challenging and involves elimination of environmental factors (such as tobacco smoke), controlling cough, desensitisation of cough pathways and control of extrapulmonary disorders. The emphasis is on treating the underlying cause. If this is not possible, then it is difficult to suppress a cough. In about half of cases a clear diagnosis cannot be determined and many people report limited, or no, effectiveness of medications.[41] In an ideal situation all tests would be performed before treatment, but this may not be cost-effective. Therefore, a balance of testing and empirical therapies is recommended, possibly starting with UACS, followed by CVA and GORD.[6]

Poorly managed chronic cough can cause complications such as vomiting, chest pain, rib fractures, urinary incontinence (in women), syncope, muscle pain, sleep disturbance and tiredness.[2] Almost all sufferers report a negative impact on quality of life including feelings of being fed up or depressed.[41] Many countries have developed cough guidelines and the main ones are published by the American College of Chest Physicians (ACCP),[5] European Respiratory Society (ERS),[6] the Chinese national guidelines on diagnosis and management of cough[42] and the Australian cough guidelines (CICADA).[4] Recommendations can vary but most highlight the need for proper diagnosis and steps for management.

Cough Variant Asthma Treatments

Cough variant asthma treatment is similar to asthma treatment. First-line treatments should include inhaled bronchodilators and ICS, and avoiding triggers.[38] These treatments usually have a good effect, especially corticosteroids because eosinophils are implicated in CVA and corticosteroids reduce eosinophilic inflammation. If these treatments are not successful, leukotriene receptor antagonists or oral corticosteroids may be used.[6] Poorly managed CVA can develop into a wheeze and if not treated with ICS, up to 40% of adults can go on to develop asthma.[32] Avoidance of allergens might also be important. Well-controlled CVA is described as few symptoms, little reliever medication use, and no night waking or activity limitation.

Upper Airways Cough Syndrome Treatments

Treatments for UACS focus on rhinosinusitis management including intranasal corticosteroids, antihistamine and anticholinergics. Decongestants may be used but are generally not recommended because their effect only lasts a few days and when stopped can lead to a worse case of rebound rhinitis. For UACS the treatment selection often relies on the underlying pathology and patient preferences.[10]

Gastro-oesophageal Reflux-related Cough Treatments

People with GORD-C should undertake diet modification and lifestyle changes, such as more exercise, as well as reducing the intake of alcohol, coffee and fatty foods that will promote weight loss.[43] In addition, they should elevate the head of their bed and avoid eating three hours before bed. In people with cough, heartburn and regurgitation, there are two approaches to treatment; one is to block the stomach acid and the other to prevent the reflux wave with drugs such as proton pump inhibitors (PPIs), H_2-receptor antagonists, alginate or antacids.[43] However, PPIs do not reduce cough in 30–50% of patients, as they may reduce the acidity but not prevent the volume of reflux. They are not recommended in people with chronic cough, without heartburn or regurgitation. More importantly, overweight people with GORD should lose weight and make lifestyle modifications to gain the most improvement.

Chronic cough may persist despite treatment in about 2.7–46% of patients.[5,38] It is referred to as chronic refractory cough and is diagnosed based on exclusion of all other types of chronic cough. Treatment of refractory cough may include speech pathology, steroids, PPIs, antibiotics or bronchodilators. Other treatments, such as over-the-counter preparations, are generally not recommended due to lack of efficacy and side effects. However, menthol may help as it suppresses cough by stimulating cold receptors.[44] Opiates are no longer advised due to limited efficacy, side effects and the potential for addiction.

Prognosis

In properly diagnosed and treated cough, resolution will be achieved in up to 90% of patients.[6] For example, in people with CVA the cough may resolve in less than eight weeks after the initiation of bronchodilators or the combination of bronchodilators and ICS.[6]

Table 1.2. Chapter Summary

Definition of chronic cough	• Cough lasting more than eight weeks; • Mostly dry or minimally productive cough; • Caused by amplification of cough reflex.
Prevalence	• Reported by 10% of adults, more common in females and the obese.
Classification	Most common causes of chronic cough: • Cough variant asthma (CVA); • Upper airways cough syndrome (UACS); • Gastro-oesophageal reflux disease-related cough (GORD-C).
Diagnosis	Based on symptoms, risk factors, aggravating factors and supplementary examinations, such as chest X-ray, spirometry, cytological analysis of blood and phlegm, 24 hours of oesophageal pH monitoring.
Management	Treatments based on underlying cause: bronchodilators and/or ICS for CVA; decongestants, antihistamines and topical nasal corticosteroids for UACS. For GORD, diet modification, lifestyle changes and PPIs for patients with heartburn or regurgitation.

In patients that don't respond to treatment or with more severe or refractory cough, more intensive treatments may be trialled, such as oral corticosteroids in the short term for cough due to asthma, prokinetic therapy or antireflux surgery for GORD. In some cases, even with proper treatment, cough may persist for up to three months. Therefore, treatment duration should continue for a reasonable time to ensure optimal effects. Other diagnostics may include high-resolution chest computed tomography (CT) scan, for suspected interstitial lung disease, or bronchoscopy for some patients, such as those that do not respond to treatment or the diagnosis remains unclear.

References

1. Brooks SM. (2011) Perspective on the human cough reflex. *Cough* **7:** 10.
2. Chung KF, Pavord ID. (2008) Prevalence, pathogenesis, and causes of chronic cough. *Lancet* **371(9621):** 1364–1374.

3. Lethbridge-Çejku M, Rose D, Vickerie J. (2006) Summary health statistics for United States adults: National Health Interview Survey, 2004. National Center for Health Statistics. *Vital Health Statistics* **10(228)**.

4. Gibson PG, Chang AB, Glasgow NJ, *et al.* (2010) CICADA: Cough in children and adults: Diagnosis and assessment. Australian cough guidelines summary statement. *Med J Aust* **192(5):** 265–271.

5. Irwin RS, Baumann MH, Bolser DC, *et al.* (2006) Diagnosis and management of cough executive summary: American College of Chest Physicians evidence-based clinical practice guidelines. *Chest* **129 (1 Suppl):** S1–S23.

6. Morice AH, Fontana GA, Sovijarvi AR, *et al.* (2004) The diagnosis and management of chronic cough. *Eur Respir J* **24(3):** 481–492.

7. Kohno S, Ishida T, Uchida Y, *et al.* (2006) The Japanese Respiratory Society guidelines for management of cough. *Respirology* **11(Suppl 4):** S135–S186.

8. Morice AH, McGarvey L, Pavord I. (2006) Recommendations for the management of cough in adults. *Thorax* **61(Suppl 1):** i1–i24.

9. Irwin RS, Madison JM. (2002) The persistently troublesome cough. *Am J Respir Crit Care Med* **165(11):** 1469–1474.

10. Irwin RS, French CL, Chang AB, Altman KW. (2018) Classification of cough as a symptom in adults and management algorithms: CHEST Guideline and Expert Panel Report. *Chest* **153(1):** 196–209.

11. Lougheed MD, Turcotte SE, Fisher T. (2012) Cough variant asthma: Lessons learned from deep inspirations. *Lung* **190(1):** 17–22.

12. Corrao WM, Braman SS, Irwin RS. (1979) Chronic cough as the sole presenting manifestation of bronchial asthma. *N Engl J Med* **300(12):** 633–637.

13. Glauser FL. (1972) Variant asthma. *Ann Allergy* **30(8):** 457–459.

14. Niimi A, Matsumoto H, Mishima M. (2009) Eosinophilic airway disorders associated with chronic cough. *Pulm Pharmacol Ther* **22(2):** 114–120.

15. Morice AH. (2002) Epidemiology of cough. *Pulm Pharmacol Ther* **15(3):** 253–259.

16. Mello CJ, Irwin RS, Curley FJ. (1996) Predictive values of the character, timing, and complications of chronic cough in diagnosing its cause. *Arch Intern Med* **156(9):** 997–1003.

17. Song WJ, Chang YS, Faruqi S, *et al.* (2015) The global epidemiology of chronic cough in adults: A systematic review and meta-analysis. *Eur Respir J* **45(5):** 1479–1481.

18. Chen RC, Lai KF, Liu CL, *et al.* (2006) [An epidemiologic study of cough in young college students in Guangzhou]. *Zhonghua Liu Xing Bing Xue Za Zhi* **27(2):** 123–126.

19. Lai K, Pan J, Chen R, *et al.* (2013) Epidemiology of cough in relation to China. *Cough* **9(1):** 18.

20. Bishwajit G, Tang S, Yaya S, Feng Z. (2017) Burden of asthma, dyspnea, and chronic cough in South Asia. *Int J Chron Obstruct Pulmon Dis* **12:** 1093–1099.

21. Zemp E, Elsasser S, Schindler C, *et al.* (1999) Long-term ambient air pollution and respiratory symptoms in adults (SAPALDIA study). The SAPALDIA Team. *Am J Respir Crit Care Med* **159(4 Pt 1):** 1257–1266.

22. Irwin RS, Curley FJ, French CL. (1990) Chronic cough: The spectrum and frequency of causes, key components of the diagnostic evaluation, and outcome of specific therapy. *Am Rev Respir Dis* **141(3):** 640–647.

23. World Health Organisation (2018). Global health estimates 2016: Disease burden by cause, age, sex, by country and by region, 2000–2016. World Health Organisation, Geneva.

24. Nurmagambetov T, Kuwahara R, Garbe P. (2018) The economic burden of asthma in the United States, 2008–2013. *Ann Am Thorac Soc* **15(3):** 348–356.

25. Accordini S, Corsico A, Cerveri I, *et al.* (2008) The socio-economic burden of asthma is substantial in Europe. *Allergy* **63(1):** 116–124.

26. Bahadori K, Doyle-Waters MM, Marra C, *et al.* (2009) Economic burden of asthma: A systematic review. *BMC Pulm Med* **9:** 24.

27. Morice AH, Jakes AD, Faruqi S, *et al.* (2014) A worldwide survey of chronic cough: A manifestation of enhanced somatosensory response. *Eur Respir J* **44(5):** 1149–1155.

28. Colak Y, Nordestgaard BG, Laursen LC, *et al.* (2017) Risk factors for chronic cough among 14,669 individuals from the general population. *Chest* **152(3):** 563–573.

29. Groneberg DA, Nowak D, Wussow A, Fischer A. (2006) Chronic cough due to occupational factors. *J Occup Med Toxicol* **1:** 3.

30. Hu ZW, Zhao YN, Cheng Y, *et al.* (2016) Living near a major road in Beijing: Association with lower lung function, airway acidification, and chronic cough. *Chin Med J* **129(18):** 2184–2190.

31. Bentayeb M, Norback D, Bednarek M, *et al.* (2015) Indoor air quality, ventilation and respiratory health in elderly residents living in nursing homes in Europe. *Eur Respir J* **45(5):** 1228–1238.

32. Niimi A. (2011) Cough and asthma. *Curr Respir Med Rev* **7(1):** 47–54.

33. Dicpinigaitis PV. (2006) Angiotensin-converting enzyme inhibitor-induced cough: ACCP evidence-based clinical practice guidelines. *Chest* **129(1 Suppl):** S169–S173.

34. Niimi A, Amitani R, Suzuki K, *et al.* (1998) Eosinophilic inflammation in cough variant asthma. *Eur Respir J* **11(5):** 1064–1069.

35. Dicpinigaitis PV. (2006) Chronic cough due to asthma: American College of Chest Physicians evidence-based clinical practice guidelines. *Chest* **129(1 Suppl):** S75–S79.

36. Niimi A, Torrego A, Nicholson AG, *et al.* (2005) Nature of airway inflammation and remodeling in chronic cough. *J Allergy Clin Immunol* **116(3):** 565–570.

37. Bucca CB, Bugiani M, Culla B, *et al.* (2011) Chronic cough and irritable larynx. *J Allergy Clin Immunol* **127(2):** 412–419.

38. Gibson PG, Vertigan AE. (2015) Management of chronic refractory cough. *BMJ* **351:** h5590.

39. Morice AH. (2010) Cough. Available from: http://www.issc.info/.

40. Lai K, Chen R, Peng W, Zhan W. (2017) Non-asthmatic eosinophilic bronchitis and its relationship with asthma. *Pulm Pharmacol Ther* **47:** 66–71.

41. Chamberlain SA, Garrod R, Douiri A, *et al.* (2015) The impact of chronic cough: A cross-sectional European survey. *Lung* **193(3):** 401–408.

42. Asthma Workgroup of the Chinese Society of Respiratory Diseases. Chinese Medicine Association. (2015) The Chinese national guidelines on diagnosis and management of cough. *Chin J Tubere Respir Dis* **39:** 323–353.

43. Kahrilas PJ, Altman KW, Chang AB, *et al.* (2016) Chronic cough due to gastroesophageal reflux in adults: CHEST Guideline and Expert Panel Report. *Chest* **150(6):** 1341–1360.

44. Morice AH, Marshall AE, Higgins KS, Grattan TJ. (1994) Effect of inhaled menthol on citric acid-induced cough in normal subjects. Thorax **49(10):** 1024–1026.

2

Chronic Cough in Chinese Medicine

OVERVIEW

Chronic cough is a common condition attributed to Lung deficiency, leading to internal damage and dysfunction of *zang fu* 脏腑. Internal pathogenic factors attack the Lungs and the Lung *qi* fails to descend, causing upward counterflow of Lung *qi* and cough. Based on Chinese medicine theory, chronic cough is characterised as a deficiency and excess condition, and treatments should distinguish weakened body resistance from pathogenic factors. This chapter summarises the knowledge of Chinese medicine for chronic cough based on recommendations from Chinese medicine guidelines and textbooks, including its aetiology, pathogenesis, syndromes and treatment with Chinese herbal medicine, acupuncture and other Chinese medicine therapies. In the Chinese medicine literature chronic cough is not routinely described as cough variant asthma, upper airways cough syndrome, or gastro-oesophageal reflux disease as it is in Western medicine. Rather, the Chinese medicine syndromes and patterns are used. Therefore, this chapter does not separate chronic cough by type.

Introduction

Cough is a pulmonary disease caused by pathogenic attack of the Lungs. It is not only a symptom but also an independent disease. Phlegm (a concept in Chinese medicine [CM] theory) is an integral part of cough. However, symptomatically cough may be dry without expectoration or wet with expectoration. In CM, chronic cough is defined by the presence of a predominant cough which lasts for a long time or there are recurrent attacks. A specific amount of time, e.g. eight weeks, as defined in Western medicine, is not mentioned in the CM diagnosis of chronic cough but clinically it is often seen in patients experiencing cough for several months. In CM nomenclature, chronic cough is known as *Jiu Ke* 久咳 (prolonged cough), *Jiu Sou* 久嗽 (enduring cough) and *Wan Ke* 顽咳 (intractable cough).[1]

The first known record of cough in the CM literature was in the *Yellow Emperor's Classic on Internal Medicine Huang Di Nei Jing, Su Wen* for the five *Zang* 黄帝内经素问·五脏生成 (published before AD 618). It says, "when you cough it means that the *qi* is stagnant in the chest and characterised as ascending *qi* in the Lung and Stomach meridian". The *Huang Di Nei Jing* 黄帝内经素问·五脏生成 systematically describes the pathogenesis, symptoms, syndrome classification and treatment for cough. *Su Wen Cough* 素问·咳论 says, "The skin is an extension of the Lungs and the evil *qi* easily invades the skin first. When you eat cold foods the stomach can become swollen and transmit the cold to the Lung meridian and the Lungs, leading to cough." This book also mentions that "five *zang* and six *fu* can all cause cough, not only the Lung". This indicates that the external pathogenic factors attacking the Lungs lead to cough, but internal dysfunction can also result in cough.

The cough terms *Jiu Ke* and *Jiu Sou* were first recorded in *Zhu Bing Yuan Hou Lun* 诸病源候论 (c. AD 610) during the Sui dynasty. The chronic cough chapter states, "A small amount of cold attacks the Lungs, which can lead to cough. If cough lasts for a long time and does not improve, it will develop into chronic cough. If the dysfunction of five viscera *zang* leads to cough and has not been effectively treated, it will spread to its corresponding *fu*. When cough has not improved for a long time, it will also affect the function of *San Jiao* 三焦, manifesting as cough, abdominal distention, and loss of appetite. The reason is that cold accumulates in the Stomach and is related to the Lung." The above indicates that doctors in the Sui dynasty paid special attention to the pathogeny of cold, documenting that the cold pathogen was often the cause of cough. Historical CM books described the pathogenesis, regular patterns and symptoms of the whole process from initial cough to chronic cough, providing a theoretical basis for future physicians to understand chronic cough in CM theory.

Aetiology and Pathogenesis

During the Ming dynasty (1369–1644), Dr. Zang Jingyue divided the causes of cough into two categories[2]: exogenous and endogenous cough. This is still used as the basic differentiation in clinical practice today. Exogenous cough is due to external contraction of six excesses invading from the mouth, nose or skin, which will lead to inability of the Lung *qi* to circulate and failing to descend. Endogenous cough is caused by dysfunction of the *zang fu*. The internal pathogenic factors attack the Lungs and vital *qi* is consumed, causing Lung *qi* to reflux and cause cough. The endogenous cough can be classified as a dysfunction of the Lung itself due to weakness of the Lung and a dysfunction of other *zang fu* affecting the Lungs. The main reason for the endogenous cough is external contraction of pathogenic factors. Cough may also be caused by inhalation of irritants. Chronic cough lasts a long time, is hard to treat and to get complete resolution, and recurs over time. Therefore, it is a mixture of pathogenic *qi* and deficient healthy *qi*.

In addition to the Lungs, chronic cough is also related to the Liver and Spleen, as well as the Kidney. Pathogens may come from outside or inside the body. Pathological factors mainly include wind, phlegm, cold and heat. Root deficiency relates to Lung deficiency, in addition to Spleen and Kidney deficiency.

Syndrome Differentiation and Treatments

The fundamental therapeutic principles of chronic cough should distinguish weakened body resistance from pathogenic factors. If there is an excess, then pathogenic factors should be eliminated to suppress the cough and prevent pathogenic factors staying in the body. If there is deficiency, treatments should tonify the healthy *qi*. If there is severe wind attacking the Lungs and stagnation of phlegm in the pharynx and throat, this is judged as an excess syndrome, and deficiency of Lung *yin*. If there is phlegm-dampness obstructing the Lungs, Stomach *qi* ascending and Liver fire attacking the Lungs it is both deficiency and excess, but excess is predominant. The treatment of chronic cough should be based on the excess and/or deficiency syndromes and the immediate needs of the patient. The focus cannot be only on relieving cough, but also dispelling the wind, dispersing the Lung *qi*, relieving sore throat, clearing the Liver, harmonising the Stomach and nourishing *yin*.

Chinese medicine treatments recommended by guidelines, expert consensus, textbooks and monographs were used in this section (Table 2.1). The references included are as follows.[3–7]

- *Chinese Internal Medicine Guidelines for Common Diseases;*
- *Guideline of Features and Advantages of Traditional Chinese Medicine;*
- *Expert Consensus of Chinese Medicine Diagnosis and Treatment of Cough;*
- *Internal Medicine of Chinese Medicine;*
- *Practical Internal Medicine of Chinese Medicine.*

Table 2.1. Summary of Chinese Herbal Medicine for Chronic Cough

Syndrome Differentiation	Treatment Principle	Formulas
Severe wind attacking the Lungs	Disperse wind and the Lung and relieve spasms to suppress cough.	Su huang zhi ke tang 苏黄止咳汤
Phlegm-dampness obstructing the Lungs	Dry dampness to resolve phlegm and regulate *qi* to suppress cough.	Er chen tang 二陈汤 combined with San zi yang qin tang 三子养亲汤
Phlegm congealing in the throat	Reduce phlegm and soothe the throat and direct *qi* downward to suppress cough.	Qing yan li qiao tang 清咽利窍汤
Stomach *qi* ascending upwards	Reverse counterflow and resolve phlegm and harmonise the Stomach and suppress cough.	Suan fu dai zhe tang 旋覆代赭汤 combined with Ban xia xie xin tang 半夏泻心汤
Liver fire attacking the Lungs	Clear heat and purge the Liver and resolve phlegm to suppress cough.	Dai ge san 黛蛤散 combined with Huang qin xie bai san 黄芩泻白散
Deficiency of Lung *yin*	Nourish *yin* and clear heat and moisten the Lungs to suppress cough.	Sha shen mai dong tang 沙参麦冬汤

The ingredients included in the formulas listed in each section are referenced to the *Zhong Yi Fang Ji Da Ci Dian* 中医方剂大辞典.[8] Note that the use of some herbs such as *ma huang* 麻黄 may be restricted in some countries. Readers are advised to comply with relevant regulations.

Chinese Herbal Medicine Treatment Based on Syndrome Differentiation

Severe Wind Attacking the Lungs

Definition: A syndrome attributable either to external wind or to *zang fu* wind; patients may have sputum or a dry cough.

Clinical manifestations: Itchy throat, coughing due to a choking sensation, dry cough without sputum or with a small amount of sputum. Symptoms may worsen at night or in the morning. If patients encounter cold and heat changes in the external environment or odours, it can lead to aggravation or recurrent cough and shortness of breath. Symptoms will occur frequently. Tongue will have a thin and white coat and pulse will be string-like.

Treatment principle: Disperse wind and the Lung; relieve spasms to suppress cough.

Formula: *Su huang zhi ke tang* 苏黄止咳汤.

Herbs: *Zhi ma huang* 炙麻黄, *zi su zi* 紫苏子, *zi su ye* 紫苏叶, *chan tui* 蝉蜕, *qian hu* 前胡, *wu wei zi* 五味子, *niu bang zi* 牛蒡子, *di long* 地龙 and *pi pa ye* 枇杷叶.

Main actions of herbs: *Zhi ma huang* 炙麻黄 and *zi su ye* 紫苏叶 diffuse the Lung to suppress cough; *wu wei zi* 五味子 and *pi pa ye* 枇杷叶 constrain the Lung to suppress cough and resolve phlegm to relieve spasm; *zi su zi* 紫苏子 and *qian hu* 前胡 regulate the *qi* movement; *di long* 地龙, *chan tui* 蝉蜕 and *niu bang zi* 牛蒡子 disperse wind and soothe the throat to relieve itch.

Phlegm-dampness Obstructing the Lungs

Definition: A syndrome that arises when dampness gathers to form phlegm. Cough is accompanied by profuse whitish expectoration and oppression in the chest associated with phlegm, heaviness and nausea.

Clinical manifestations: Cough with profuse sputum and heavy turbid voice. Cough is due to excessive phlegm, so cough will be relieved when phlegm is reduced. Phlegm is white and sticky, or thick or thin. Cough and phlegm often increase in the morning or after meals. Accompanying symptoms include chest tightness, abdominal distention, loss of appetite, weakness and loose stools. There is also a white and shiny tongue coat and soggy and slippery pulse.

Treatment principle: Dry dampness to resolve phlegm and regulate *qi* to suppress cough.

Formulas: *Er chen tang* 二陈汤 combined with *San zi yang qin tang* 三子养亲汤.

Herbs: *Fa ban xia* 法半夏, *ju hong* 橘红, *fu ling* 茯苓, *zhi gan cao* 炙甘草, *cang zhu* 苍术, *hou pu* 厚朴, *bai jie zi* 白芥子, *lai fu zi* 莱菔子 and *zi su zi* 紫苏子.

Main actions of herbs: *Fa ban xia* 法半夏 and *ju hong* 橘红 dry dampness to resolve phlegm and regulate *qi* movement to suppress cough; *cang zhu* 苍术 and *hou pu* 厚朴 strengthen the power of drying dampness to resolve phlegm; *bai jie zi* 白芥子, *lai fu zi* 莱菔子 and *zi su zi* 紫苏子 warm the Lung to resolve the phlegm and direct *qi* downward to suppress cough; *zhi gan cao* 炙甘草 fortifies the Spleen to harmonise the middle energiser and harmonise the herbs.

Phlegm Congealing in the Throat

Definition: A syndrome marked by discomfort and a sensation of a foreign body present in the throat. Self-perception of phlegm stimulation causes coughing, glossy tongue coating and fine, string-like slippery pulse.

Clinical manifestations: Sudden attacks, intensification or persistent cough mainly appear during the day which decreases in the evening. There may also be an itchy sensation in the throat and an uncomfortable sensation of phlegm congealing in the throat. Slightly red tongue body with white, thin and mild glossy tongue coat, fine and slippery pulse or fine, string-like and slippery pulse.

Treatment principle: Reduce phlegm and soothe the throat, direct *qi* downward to suppress cough.

Formula: *Qing yan li qiao tang* 清咽利窍汤.

Herbs: *Zi su ye* 紫苏叶, *bo he* 薄荷, *jie geng* 桔梗, *jing jie* 荆芥, *mu hu die* 木蝴蝶, *niu bang zi* 牛蒡子, *tao ren* 桃仁, *bai bu* 百部, *she gan* 射干, *xin yi hua* 辛夷花, *cang er zi* 苍耳子 and *sheng gan cao* 生甘草.

Main actions of herbs: *Zi su ye* 紫苏叶 regulates *qi* to relieve Liver *qi* depression and regulates *qi* movement; *bo he* 薄荷 and *jing jie* 荆芥 disperse wind to dispel the pathogen; *jie geng* 桔梗 diffuses the Lung to dispel phlegm and direct the herbs up to Lungs; *mu hu die* 木蝴蝶 and *niu bang zi* 牛蒡子 clear the heat to soothe the throat and relieve itch to suppress cough; *bai bu* 百部 moistens the Lung to direct *qi* downward and resolve phlegm to suppress cough; *tao ren* 桃仁 activates blood and resolves stasis; *cang er zi* 苍耳子 and *xin yi hua* 辛夷花 diffuse the nose; *she gan* 射干 dispels the phlegm to soothe the throat and resolve stasis to eliminate masses; *sheng gan cao* 生甘草 harmonises all medicinal herbs.

Stomach *Qi* Ascending Upwards

Definition: Upward ascent of Stomach *qi* causes the Lung to fail to disperse and descend *qi* and adversely ascend *qi*. The pathogenic manifestations include cough, belching, hiccups, acid regurgitation and vomiting.

Clinical manifestations: Sudden attack or intensified cough and shortness of breath; symptoms may worsen after lying flat or overeating. Easy to suffer from abdominal discomfort, accompanied with acid regurgitation, belching, gastric stuffiness and scorching pain, red tongue with white, yellow and slimy coat, and string-like and slippery pulse.

Treatment principle: Reverse upward counterflow and resolve phlegm, harmonise the stomach and suppress cough.

Formulas: *Xuan fu dai zhe tang* 旋覆代赭汤 combined with *Ban xia xie xin tang* 半夏泻心汤.

Herbs: *Xuan fu hua* 旋覆花, *dai zhe shi* 代赭石, *fa ban xia* 法半夏, *gan jiang* 干姜, *huang lian* 黄连, *huang qin* 黄芩, *da zao* 大枣, *dang shen* 党参, *pi pa ye* 枇杷叶, *duan wa len* 煅瓦楞 and *zhi gan cao* 炙甘草.

Main actions of herbs: *Xuan fu hua* 旋覆花 and *dai zhe shi* 代赭石 direct *qi* downward to resolve phlegm and stop vomiting; *fa ban xia* 法半夏 dispels phlegm to dissipate binds and direct *qi* downward to harmonise the Stomach; *gan jiang* 干姜 warms the middle to dissipate cold; *huang lian* 黄连 and *huang qin* 黄芩 discharge heat to alleviate stuffiness; *dang shen* 党参 and *da zao* 大枣 tonify *qi* and fortify the Spleen; *pi pa ye* 枇杷叶 clears the Lung heat, harmonises the Stomach and directs *qi* downwards to resolve phlegm; *duan wa len* 煅瓦楞 eliminates phlegm, resolves stasis, softens hardness and dissipates binds; *zhi gan cao* 炙甘草 tonifies the Spleen and harmonises the middle and other herbs.

Liver Fire Attacking the Lungs

Definition: A syndrome marked by bitter taste in the mouth, dizziness, red eyes, irritability, easily angered disposition, moving pain in the chest and hypochondriac region, cough with thick expectoration or haemoptysis, red tongue body and rapid, tight string-like pulse.

Clinical manifestations: Sudden attack, intensified cough or severe cough accompanied by shortness of breath and reddish complexion. Dry throat, bitter taste in the mouth, a small amount of sticky phlegm congealed in the throat that is difficult to bring up, sometimes appearing with small white clumps of phlegm. Symptoms are associated with mood swings and the cough may aggravate chest pain. Red tongue body or margins of the tongue with thin, yellow and dry coat and string-like and rapid pulse.

Treatment principle: Clear heat and Liver and resolve phlegm to suppress cough.

Formulas: *Dai ge san* 黛蛤散 combined with *Huang qin xie bai san* 黄芩泻白散.

Herbs: *Qing dai* 青黛, *hai ge ke* 海蛤壳, *sang bai pi* 桑白皮, *di gu pi* 地骨皮, *huang qin* 黄芩, *shan zhi zi* 山栀子, *mu dan pi* 牡丹皮, *zi su zi* 紫苏子, *zhu ru* 竹茹, *pi pa ye* 枇杷叶 and *gan cao* 甘草.

Main actions of herbs: *Qing dai* 青黛 and *hai ge ke* 海蛤壳 clear the Liver and resolve phlegm; *sang bai pi* 桑白皮, *di gu pi* 地骨皮 and *huang qin* 黄芩 clear and purge the Lung heat; *shan zhi zi* 山栀子 and *mu dan pi* 牡丹皮 clear and purge the Liver fire; *zi su zi* 紫苏子, *zhu ru* 竹茹 and *pi pa ye* 枇杷叶 direct *qi* downward; *gan cao* 甘草 harmonises the middle, nourishes the Stomach and harmonises other herbs. These formulas can purge the Lung but will not injure the Spleen and Stomach.

Deficiency of Lung *Yin*

Definition: A syndrome attributed to *yin* deficiency of the Lung with endogenous heat, manifesting as unproductive cough, afternoon fever, night sweating, flushed cheeks, dry throat, red and dry tongue, and rapid fine pulse.

Clinical manifestations: Dry cough with a transient and hurried voice, a small amount of white and slimy phlegm, sometimes streaked with blood. Coughing can also lead to hoarseness. Dry mouth and throat, accompanied by afternoon fever, flushed cheeks and lassitude of spirit. Red tongue body with a fine coat and fine and rapid pulse.

Treatment principle: Nourish *yin* and clear heat and moisten the Lung to suppress cough.

Formula: *Sha shen mai dong tang* 沙参麦冬汤.

Herbs: *Bei sha shen* 北沙参, *mai dong* 麦冬, *yu zhu* 玉竹, *tian hua fen* 天花粉, *sang ye* 桑叶, *bai he* 百合, *chuan bei mu* 川贝母 and *gan cao* 甘草.

Main actions of herbs: *Bei sha shen* 北沙参 and *mai dong* 麦冬 clear and nourish the Lung and Stomach; *yu zhu* 玉竹 and *tian hua fen* 天花粉 clear heat to nourish *yin* and engender fluid to suppress thirst; *sang ye* 桑叶 clears the Lung heat and moistens dryness; *bai he* 百合 and *chuan bei mu* 川贝母 nourish *yin* to moisten the Lung, relieve cough and resolve phlegm; *gan cao* 甘草 harmonises all herbs.

Single Herb Formula

Chuan bei 川贝: Core one pear then put 5g of *chuan bei* 川贝 powder and a small amount of crystal sugar into the pear; stew together and eat. It can moisten the Lung to nourish *yin* and resolve phlegm to suppress cough. Suitable for deficiency of Lung *yin*.

Bai he 百合: Take 30g of decocted *bai he* 百合 to nourish *yin* and moisten the Lung. Suitable for deficiency of Lung *yin*.

Acupuncture Therapy

The main acupuncture points are BL13 *Feishu* 肺俞, LU1 *Zhongfu* 中府, LU7 *Lieque* 列缺 and LU9 *Taiyuan* 太渊.[3] Based on syndrome differentiation, the following points can be used:

- Stomach *qi* ascending upwards: add ST36 *Zusanli* 足三里, PC6 *Neiguan* 内关 and ST40 *Fenglong* 丰隆;
- Liver fire attacking the Lungs: add LR2 *Xingjian* 行间 and LU10 *Yuji* 鱼际;
- Deficiency of Lung *yin*: Add BL43 *Gaohuang* 膏肓 and KI3 *Taixi* 太溪.

For excess syndromes use a reducing method and for deficiency syndromes use reinforcing methods.

Moxibustion can also be used on the following points: GV14 *Dazhui* 大椎, BL13 *Feishu* 肺俞 (or BL12 *Fengmen* 风门) and BL43 *Gao huang* 膏肓. A 0.5 cm cone of moxibustion can be used once every three to five days; repeat five times to make one course of treatment. Moxa sticks can also be used daily; use for five to ten minutes on each point until the skin is slightly red.

Other Management Strategies

Lifestyle Modification

Patients with chronic cough should keep warm and prevent catching a cold when the temperature changes. Patients should pay attention to air circulation in bedrooms and during sleep. Irritant gases, dust and pollen should be avoided. Diet should be light and nourishing and raw, cold, fatty and spicy foods, as well as seafood, should be avoided. Patients should abstain from tobacco and alcohol. Patients should keep their mood calm and avoid influences that put them in a bad mood. In addition, they should pay attention to balancing work and rest to prevent excessive tiredness.

Physical Exercise

Patients with chronic cough should strengthen themselves by participating in physical exercise to improve their constitution. According to their physical condition, patients need to make a moderate, sustainable and long-term exercise plan, and engage in activities such as *ba duan jin* 八段锦, *taichi* 太极, *qigong* 气功 and jogging. These physical exercises can improve lung function, strengthen physique and improve disease resistance.

Herbal Prevention

Other herbal medicines can be taken depending on syndrome differentiation (see Table 2.1); for example, patients who are prone to sweating and common cold and cough recurrence can take *Yu ping feng san* 玉屏风散 or *Bu zhong yi qi tang* 补中益气汤. Patients with Lung *yin* deficiency can use *Sheng mai yin* 生脉饮.

References

1. 中华医学会呼吸病学分会哮喘学组. (2016) 咳嗽的诊断与治疗指南 2015. 中华结核和呼吸杂志. **39(5):** 323–354.
2. 张介宾. (2016) 景岳全书. 北京: 中国医药科技出版社.
3. 中华中医药学会内科分会肺系病专业委员会. (2011) 咳嗽中医诊疗专家共识意见 (2011版). 中医杂志. **52(10):** 896–899.
4. 吴勉华, 王新月. (2013) 全国中医药行业高等教育"十二五"规划教材·中医内科学. 北京: 中国中医药出版社.
5. 周仲瑛. (2012) 薛博瑜. 实用中医内科学·肺系病证. 第1版. 北京: 中国中医药出版社.
6. 罗云坚, 孙塑伦. (2008) 中医临床治疗特色与优势指南. 北京: 人民卫生出版社.
7. 中华中医药学会. (2008) 中医内科常见病诊疗指南 中医疾病部分. 北京: 中国中医药出版社.
8. 彭怀仁. (1997) 中医方剂大辞典. 北京: 人民卫生出版社.

3

Classical Chinese Medicine Literature

OVERVIEW

The classical Chinese medicine literature provides a valuable resource of information for prevention and management of conditions and diseases. This chapter describes the findings of a systematic evaluation of the classical Chinese medicine literature for chronic cough. The comprehensive search was conducted on the *Zhong Hua Yi Dian* 中华医典, one of the largest digital collections of medical books available. A total of 436 citations describing the management of chronic cough were identified. Aetiology and pathogenesis, treatments with Chinese herbal medicine, acupuncture and other Chinese medicine therapies for chronic cough were analysed and summarised.

Introduction

The first known written records of Chinese medicine (CM) in professional practice date back as early as the Spring and Autumn (770–476 BC) and Warring states (474–221 BC) periods in ancient China.[1] Over thousands of years clinical doctors have documented precious information and knowledge of the aetiology, pathogenesis, symptoms, syndromes and clinical management of various diseases in the CM classical literature. This literature has contributed to the contemporary knowledge and treatment of chronic cough.

In classical CM literature, chronic cough was usually described as the terms *jiu ke* 久咳 and *jiu sou* 久嗽 under the disease category of *ke sou* 咳嗽 (cough). Chronic cough could appear as an individual disease or an accompanying symptom of other diseases. About 1,500 to 2,000 years ago, ancient CM practitioners started documenting the aetiology and pathogenesis of cough in the book *Yellow Emperor's Classic on Internal Medicine Huang Di Nei Jing* 黄帝内经. In the *Su Wen Ke Lun Pian* 素问咳论篇 section, the author further pointed out that chronic cough related to the five viscera *zang* 脏, affecting the six bowels *fu* 腑 (五脏之久咳, 乃移于六腑), inducing symptoms. Over the long history of the clinical management of chronic cough, the CM theory of chronic cough and treatment methods have been established systematically. Some of this experience has contributed to the contemporary knowledge of chronic cough. However, comprehensively summarising and evaluating the historical CM treatment for chronic cough remains a challenge due to the large number of classical books. In order to address this, the digital *Zhong Hua Yi Dian* (ZHYD) 中华医典 CD-ROM, which includes more than 1,000 CM medical books, was developed and used in this analysis.[2] This collection is the largest currently available and is representative of other large collections of the classical and pre-modern CM literature,[3–4] making it convenient to systematically search and analyse CM books dating back thousands of years.

Search Terms

To find citations from the classical literature, search terms that describe chronic cough in traditional Chinese language needed to be identified. To do this, a group of CM textbooks, professional books and guidelines on chronic cough was accessed to identify the relevant search terms, including the following[5–8]:

- Professional Committee of Pulmonary Diseases, Internal Medicine Branch, Chinese Society of Traditional Chinese Medicine. Experts Consensus of Chinese Medicine Diagnosis and Treatment of Cough.
- Internal Medicine of Chinese Medicine; Beijing: China Press of Traditional Chinese Medicine.
- National Standard Application: Routine Diagnosis and Treatment of Diseases in Internal Medicine of Traditional Chinese Medicine; Hunan: Hunan Science and Technology Press.
- Internal Medicine of Chinese Medicine; Beijing: People's Medical Publishing House.

Three search terms were selected in consultation with CM specialists and experts, including *jiu ke* 久咳, *jiu sou* 久嗽 and *tan yin ke sou* 痰饮咳嗽. The terms *jiu ke* 久咳 and *jiu sou* 久嗽 directly describe 'chronic cough' and were selected because they are used in both classical and contemporary CM literature. *Tan yin ke sou* 痰饮咳嗽 describes 'cough with sputum'. It was selected because it describes the symptoms that are typically seen during the course of chronic cough, not because it describes chronic cough itself.

Procedures for Search, Data Coding and Data Analysis

The three included search terms (*jiu ke* 久咳, *jiu sou* 久嗽 and *tan yin ke sou* 痰饮咳嗽) were then entered into the ZHYD database search fields separately. Both headings and full-text searches were conducted for each term and the search results were exported to spreadsheets for cleaning and coding. A 'citation' was defined as a distinct passage of text referring to one or more of the search terms. Duplicate citations identified by different search terms were removed from the dataset. Citations published after 1949 were also removed because they are not considered to be 'classical' Chinese literature; rather, they are 'modern' Chinese literature.

After duplicate removal, inclusion and exclusion criteria were applied to determine the eligibility of each citation in terms of its likelihood of describing chronic cough. Citations that mentioned chronic cough as the only, or the main, symptom were included. Citations that were judged to be other diseases or conditions, such as haemoptysis, tuberculosis and asthma, were excluded. Citations that mentioned children were also excluded. The full exclusion criteria included the following:

- Citations that mentioned any other disease names or conditions besides chronic cough, such as *tuo xue* 唾血 (haemoptysis), *lao zhai* 痨瘵 (tuberculosis), *fei lao* 肺痨 (tuberculosis), *fei zhang* 肺胀 (pulmonary emphysema or core pulmonale), *fei wei* 肺痿 (pulmonary interstitial fibrosis), *chuan zheng* 喘证 (asthma or chronic obstructive pulmonary disease) or *fei yong* 肺痈 (pulmonary abscess);
- Citations that mentioned any symptom which might refer to another disease or condition such as coughing pus or blood,

coughing and dyspnoea in semi-reclining position, asthma and shortness of breath, coughing with wheezing sound, oedema and feeling fever steaming from the bones;

• Citations that mentioned children.

All relevant citations were reviewed to identify the best descriptions of chronic cough and its aetiology and/or pathogenesis. Relevant citations which did not include a treatment for chronic cough were excluded from further analysis. The final dataset included citations with chronic cough as the main symptom and described a CM treatment such as Chinese herbal medicine (CHM), acupuncture and related therapies, or other CM therapies for example, *tai chi* or *qigong*. When a citation referred to multiple treatments, each treatment was considered as a separate citation for calculation of formulas, herbs or acupuncture points. For the identified Chinese herbal formulas that did not specify ingredients, the ingredients were sourced from the same formula in the same book if possible.

Included citations were grouped into one of three categories according to the CM intervention for further analysis including (1) Chinese herbal medicine, (2) acupuncture, and (3) other CM therapies. The main data generated from the classical literature are the common herbs and acupuncture treatments, and how frequently they were used over time.

Search Results

The search terms were found in a total of 1,300 citations (Table 3.1). *Jiu sou* 久嗽 yielded the highest number of hits (626 instances,

Table 3.1. Terms Used to Identify Classical Literature Citations and Hit Frequency

Search Terms of Chronic Cough in Pinyin	Search Terms of Chronic Cough in Chinese	English Translation	Total Hit Frequency, *n* (%)
Jiu sou	久嗽	Chronic cough	626 (48.2)
Tan yin ke sou	痰饮咳嗽	Cough with sputum	446 (34.3)
Jiu ke	久咳	Chronic cough	228 (17.5)

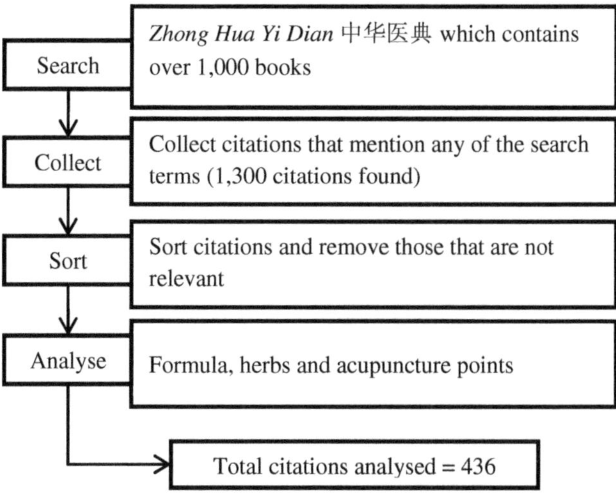

Fig. 3.1. Flow diagram of classical literature citations.

48.2%), followed by *tan yin ke sou* 痰饮咳嗽 and *jiu ke* 久咳, 446 and 228, respectively.

Citations Related to Chronic Cough

After duplicate removal, the citations were then reviewed for eligibility according to the inclusion and exclusion criteria as mentioned above. A total of 436 citations met the criteria and were related to chronic cough (Fig. 3.1). All of the included citations were also reviewed to identify and synthesise the aetiological and pathogenic details, and CM interventions were extracted, coded and further analysed.

Of the 436 citations, 355 (81.4%) described CHM treatments, 29 (6.7%) mentioned acupuncture and/or moxibustion therapies, while 52 (11.9%) described other CM therapies such as inhaling herbal smoke therapy for treating chronic cough.

Definitions of the Condition and Aetiology

Chronic cough was mentioned in many classical literature citations, dating from the Warring States period (474–221 BC). Chronic cough appeared as an individual symptom, or alongside other symptoms, and was related to a variety of *zang* and *fu* disorders. One of the earliest citations was from the Warring States period as cited in the book *Huang Di Nei Jing Su Wen* 黄帝内经素问 (before AD 618); it stated "the five viscera *zang* and six bowels *fu* can all cause a person to cough, not only the Lung" (五脏六腑皆能令人咳, 非独肺也).

An example of a later citation is from the book *Tai Yi Yuan Mi Cang Gao Dan Wan San Fang Ji* 太医院秘藏膏丹丸散方剂 (c. 1911). It stated that the herbal formula *Shen su li fei wan* 参苏理肺丸 could be used to treat diseases related to the Lung meridian. Patients with long-term disease, coughing day and night and in all seasons, runny nose and coughing up sputum, weak limbs and fatigue would benefit from this formula (参苏理肺丸, 此丸专治肺经不清 … 及经年旧病, 咳嗽昼夜不安, 春秋举发, 鼻流清涕, 痰涎壅盛, 四肢无力, 身体困倦).

Due to the nature of the classical literature and the importance of *zang fu,* the following section is separated by the various aetiologies and pathologies for chronic cough.

Chronic Cough Related to the Lungs

In CM theory, the Lungs govern *qi* and respiration. Any pathogen that affects the Lungs may cause disordered diffusion of Lung *qi* and manifest as chronic cough. The aetiology and pathogenesis of chronic cough and its association with the Lungs have been discussed in depth in classical literature. Fire (heat) was identified as the most frequently mentioned pathogenic factor causing chronic cough. Dr. Wu Yi Luo in the Qing dynasty discussed the aetiology and treatment principles for chronic cough in his book *Cheng Fang Qie Yong* 成方切用 (c. 1761). He stated that 'Lung is the umbrella of the five viscera, and it governs *qi* and expresses voice and sound' (肺为五脏华盖 … 为气之主, 而出声也). 'When the Lung is harmed by fire, *qi* refluxes and causes cough' (肺受火伤, 则气逆而为咳). Dr. Sun Yi Kui in the book *Chi Shui Xuan Zhu* 赤水玄珠, published in the Ming dynasty (c. 1573), held a similar view and stated that 'excessive heat in the upper energiser could cause chronic cough with sputum, oppression and fullness of the chest (日久痰嗽, 胸膈不利, 上焦多热). Stagnant heat affecting Lung *qi* could also induce chronic cough with nasal drip and sputum (c.1117, *Sheng Ji Zong Lu* 圣济总录, '肺气壅热, 久嗽涕唾多').

Other pathogenic factors affecting the Lungs were also mentioned in classical literature. In *Shi Fang Miao Yong* 时方妙用 (c. 1803) Dr. Chen Xiu Yuan pointed out that dryness could be a factor; he wrote, 'If patients are suffering from chronic cough, Lung could be affected by dryness. In this situation, excessive cough could induce all kinds of fire and harm the Lungs' (若久嗽之人, 肺必干燥, 且以多咳而牵引诸火而刑金).

Wu Zhi Wang in his book *Ji Yang Gang Mu* 济阳纲目 (c. 1626) detailed chronic cough caused by deficient cold. It says, '*Ren shen kuan hua gao* 人参款花膏 could be used to treat deficiency cold affecting the Lungs, with the symptoms of chronic cough, oppression and fullness of the throat, chest and abdomen, coughing sputum, nausea, back pain, and fatigue' (人参款化膏, 治肺受虚寒, 久嗽不已, 咽膈满闷, 咳嗽痰涎, 呕逆恶心, 腹胁胀满, 腰背倦痛). In this book, he also stated that accumulated phlegm in the Lungs could be one factor causing chronic cough, describing accumulated phlegm as sticky gum that blocks the *qi* diffusion (久嗽乃痰积久留肺脘, 粘滞如胶, 不能升降).

Chronic Cough Related to the Spleen and Stomach

In the identified classical literature citations, chronic cough could be caused by dysfunction and diseases in the middle energiser. Spleen and Stomach were mentioned as being closely related to the cause of chronic cough. In CM theory, the Spleen and Stomach carry the function of transportation and transformation of food and drink. When the normal function of the Spleen and Stomach weakens, internal phlegm arises and affects the Lungs, causing cough. The descriptions from classical literature were consistent with contemporary CM theory.

In the book *Cheng Fang Qie Yong* 成方切用 (c. 1761), the author stated that 'if there is dampness retained by the Spleen, phlegm could be produced and cause cough' (脾有停湿, 则生痰而作嗽). While in the book *Sheng Ji Zong Lu* 圣济总录 (c. 1117), the author stated that 'phlegm accumulation caused by deficient Stomach could be another factor that induces chronic cough, and there will be fullness in the abdomen and poor appetite' (久咳传三焦, 腹满不思饮食, 及胃虚有痰). This book also stated that disharmony of Lung and Stomach could cause chronic cough and could be treated by *E jiao san fang* 阿胶散方 (治肺胃不调, 久咳不瘥, 阿胶散方). In some cases, dryness could also cause damage to the Lung and Stomach *yin* and may induce chronic fever alongside chronic cough. This could be treated by modified *Sha shen mai dong tang* 沙参麦冬汤 (*Ben Cao Jian Yao Fang* 本草简要方, c. 1938, '沙参麦冬汤, 治燥伤肺胃阴分, 或热或咳. 久热, 久咳者加地骨皮三钱').

Chronic Cough Related to the Kidneys

A few classical literature citations mentioned that the Kidney could cause chronic cough. In the book, *Pu Ji Fang* 普济方 (c. 1406), the author stated that '*Zhen wu tang* 真武汤 can be used to treat Kidney *yin* syndrome. In this syndrome, *yin* and internal cold induce cough. The citation describes that elderly patients with *qi* deficiency and chronic cough can be treated with *Zhen wu tang* 真武汤 formula' (真武汤, 治少阴肾证, 水饮与里寒合而作嗽, 腹痛下. 凡年高气弱。久嗽通用). Dr. Zou Cun Gan, in his book *Wai Zhi Shou Shi Fang* 外治寿世方 (published in 1877), described a topical treatment that sends *qi* back to Kidney to treat chronic cough, suggesting insecurity of Kidney *qi* could be one factor that causes chronic cough (久嗽不止, 罂粟壳末或五倍子末, 掺膏贴脐上, 纳气归肾自止).

It is generally recognised that diseases of the Liver could also lead to chronic cough. However, in the included citations, no direct evidence of chronic cough related to Liver was identified. One possible reason might be that the relevant description related to the Liver were in the general cough group of citations that had been excluded from analysis.

Chinese Herbal Medicine

The 355 citations describing CHM treatments were identified in 64 books. *Pu Ji Fang* 普济方 (c. 1406) was the book that yielded the largest number of citations (*n* = 91). Other books with many citations included *Ji Yang Gang Mu* 济阳纲目 (c. 1626; *n* = 30), *Yan Fang Xin Bian* 验方新编 (c. 1846; *n* = 23) and *Sheng Ji Zong Lu* 圣济总录 (c. 1117; *n* = 21).

Frequency of Treatment Citations by Dynasty

The included CHM citations were obtained from the classical literature published from the Dong Jing 东晋 period (c. 317–420 BC) to Ming Guo 民国/Republic of China (1912–1949). The majority of citations (75%) were published in the Ming dynasty (c. 1369–1644) and the Qing dynasty (c. 1645–1911) (Table 3.2). The earliest citation with CHM treatment was from *Zhou Hou Bei Ji Fang* 肘后备急方 (c. AD 363), which was obtained by the search term *jiu sou* 久嗽. It mentioned the formula *Jin su wan* 金粟丸 for managing chronic cough. The formula preparation and administration methods were also detailed in this citation. The most recent citation was from the book *Ben Cao Jian Yao Fang* 本草简要方 published in the Ming Guo period (c. 1938). The aetiology and pathogenesis of chronic cough were described alongside the formulas *Sha shen mai dong tang* 沙参麦冬汤, *Zi wan gao* 紫菀膏 and *Ma bo wan* 马勃丸. This citation was typical of the more recent citations that recommend treatments based on syndrome differentia-tion, whereas earlier citations only describe the treatment of symptoms.

Table 3.2. Dynastic Distribution of Treatment Citations

Dynasty	No. of Treatment Citations
Before Tang dynasty (before 618)	4
Tang and 5 dynasties (618–960)	19
Song and Jin dynasties (961–1271)	55
Yuan dynasty (1272–1368)	4
Ming dynasty (1369–1644)	171
Qing dynasty (1645–1911)	96
Ming Guo/Republic of China (1912–1949)	6
Total	355

Treatment with Chinese Herbal Medicine

All CHM treatments were taken orally, and most were described as a formula with multiple herbal ingredients ($n = 203$, 57.2%), while 115 citations (32.4%) included multiple herbal ingredients but no formula name. A small number of citations described the use of single herbs for chronic cough ($n = 39$, 11.0%).

Most Frequent Formulas in Citations Related to Chronic Cough

Of the 203 named formulas, 13 were described in three or more citations and are presented in Table 3.3. Herbal ingredients were

Table 3.3. Most Frequent Oral Formulas in Citations Related to Chronic Cough

Formula Name	Herb Ingredients	Number of Citations (*n*)
E jiao san 阿胶散	*E jiao* 阿胶, *ren shen* 人参, *xing ren* 杏仁, *gan cao* 甘草, *huang qi* 黄芪, *zi wan* 紫菀, *jie geng* 桔梗 and *sang bai pi* 桑白皮 (*Sheng Ji Zong Lu* 圣济总录, c. 1117)	9
Bei mu tang 贝母汤	*Bei mu* 贝母, *huang qin* 黄芩, *gan jiang* 干姜, *chen pi* 陈皮, *wu wei zi* 五味子, *sang bai pi* 桑白皮, *ban xia* 半夏, *chai hu* 柴胡, *gui zhi* 桂枝, *mu xiang* 木香, *gan cao* 甘草, *xing ren* 杏仁 and *sheng jiang* 生姜 (*Pu Ji Fang* 普济方, c. 1406)	5
Bu fei tang 补肺汤	*E jiao* 阿胶, *su zi* 苏子, *jie geng* 桔梗, *ban xia* 半夏, *gan cao* 甘草, *kuan dong hua* 款冬花, *zi wan* 紫菀, *xi xin* 细辛, *xing ren* 杏仁, *chen pi* 陈皮, *sang bai pi* 桑白皮, *qing pi* 青皮, *sha ren* 砂仁, *wu wei zi* 五味子, *shi chang pu* 石菖蒲, *cao guo* 草果, *sheng jiang* 生姜 and *zi su* 紫苏 (*Ren Zhai Zhi Zhi Fang Lun* 仁斋直指方论, c. 1264)	5
Ge jie wan 蛤蚧丸	*Ge jie* 蛤蚧, *ren shen* 人参, *ban xia* 半夏, *xing ren* 杏仁, *gua lou* 瓜蒌, *e jiao* 阿胶, *qing pi* 青皮, *da zao* 大枣 and *feng mi* 蜂蜜 (*Sheng Ji Zong Lu* 圣济总录, c. 1117)	5

Table 3.3.   (*Continued*)

Formula Name	Herb Ingredients	Number of Citations (*n*)
Zi wan san 紫菀散	*Zi wan* 紫菀, *kuan dong hua* 款冬花 and *sheng jiang* 生姜 (*Tai Ping Sheng Hui Fang* 太平圣惠方, c. 992)	5
Bei mu wan 贝母丸	*Bei mu* 贝母, *kuan dong hua* 款冬花, *zi wan* 紫菀, *feng mi* 蜂蜜 and *sheng jiang* 生姜 (*Sheng Ji Zong Lu* 圣济总录, c. 1117)	3
He zi yin 诃子饮	*He zi* 诃子, *xing ren* 杏仁, *tong cao* 通草 and *sheng jiang* 生姜 (*Pu Ji Fang* 普济方, c. 1406)	3
Jin su wan 金粟丸	*Ci huang* 雌黄, *ji xiao he zi* 济小合子, *chi shi zhi* 赤石脂 and *gan cao* 甘草 (*Zhou Hou Bei Ji Fang* 肘后备急方, c. 363)	3
Jiu sou wan zi 久嗽丸子	*Hai ge ke* 海蛤壳, *dan nan xing* 胆南星, *xing ren* 杏仁, *he zi* 诃子, *qing dai* 青黛, *zao jiao* 皂角 and *sheng jiang* 生姜 (*Yi Xue Gang Mu* 医学纲目, c. 1565)	3
Ren shen kuan hua gao 人参款花膏	*Ren shen* 人参, *kuan dong hua* 款冬花, *wu wei zi* 五味子, *zi wan* 紫菀, *sang bai pi* 桑白皮, *mai dong* 麦冬, *feng mi* 蜂蜜 and *sheng jiang* 生姜 (*Ji Yang Gang Mu* 济阳纲目, c. 1626)	3
Zhi ke tang 枳壳汤	*Zhi ke* 枳壳, *jie geng* 桔梗 and *huang qin* 黄芩 (*Yi Xue Gang Mu* 医学纲目, c. 1565)	3
Zhou fei wan 皱肺丸	*Kuan dong hua* 款冬花, *ren shen* 人参, *wu wei zi* 五味子, *gui zhi* 桂枝, *zi wan* 紫菀, *bai shi ying* 白石英, *zhong ru fen* 钟乳粉, *yang fei* 羊肺 and *xing ren* 杏仁 (*Shi Zhai Bai Yi Xuan Fang* 是斋百一选方, c. 1196)	3
Zi wan wan 紫菀丸	*Zi wan* 紫菀, *kuan dong hua* 款冬花, *bai qian* 白前, *ren shen* 人参, *ting li zi* 葶苈子, *wu mei* 乌梅, *ying su* 罂粟, *feng mi* 蜂蜜 and *sheng jiang* 生姜 (*Pu Ji Fang* 普济方, c. 1406)	3

(1) Formula ingredients are based on the earliest book within the group of included citations. (2) Formulas with the same name can vary in their ingredients and the same combination of ingredients may have different names. In this data, formulas with the same name that have variations in a few ingredients are grouped together. Also, formulas with the same ingredients but different names have been grouped together. (3) The use of some herbs/ingredients may be restricted in some countries. For example, herbs such as *xi xin* 细辛, *chi shi zhi* 赤石脂 and *ci huang* 雌黄 can be toxic. Readers are advised to comply with relevant regulations.

obtained from the earliest citation if variants were seen under the same formula name.

E jiao san 阿胶散 was the most frequently described formula to treat chronic cough. The earliest citation mentioned *E jiao san* 阿胶散 in the book *Sheng ji zong lu* 圣济总录 (c. 1117). Herbal ingredients in the formula tonify *qi* and *yin*, supress cough and resolve phlegm. Most of the other frequently cited formulas had a similar function to suppress cough and resolve phlegm. The functions of the most frequent formulas were categorised as the following:

- Moisten the Lung to suppress cough (*E jiao san* 阿胶散, *Ga jie wan* 蛤蚧丸, *Bei mu wan* 贝母丸, *Zhou fei wan* 皱肺丸 and *Ren shen kuan hua gao* 人参款花膏);
- Constrain the Lung to suppress cough (*He zi yin* 诃子饮 and *Jin su wan* 金粟丸);
- Clear heat and resolve phlegm (*Jiu sou wan zi* 久嗽丸子);
- Regulate *qi* to suppress cough (*Bei mu wan* 贝母丸 and *Zhi ke tang* 枳壳汤); or
- Tonify *qi* and *yin*, supress cough and resolve phlegm (*E jiao san* 阿胶散, *Ren shen kuan hua gao* 人参款花膏 and *Zi wan san* 紫菀散).

Most Frequent Herbs in Citations Related to Chronic Cough

The 355 CHM treatments were further analysed for herb frequency. A total of 263 different herbal ingredients were identified from the included citations. The most frequently cited herbs were *sheng jiang* 生姜, *feng mi* 蜂蜜, *gan cao* 甘草, *kuan dong hua* 款冬花 and *xing ren* 杏仁 (Table 3.4).

Similar with the functions of the most frequently cited formulas, the herbs also supressed cough and resolved phlegm. A total of seven categories of herbs were identified, including herbs that do the following:

- Tonify *yin* and moisten the Lung to suppress cough, such as *feng mi* 蜂蜜 and *e jiao* 阿胶;
- Moisten the Lung and direct *qi* downward to supress cough and resolve phlegm, such as *kuan dong hua* 款冬花 and *zi wan* 紫菀;

Table 3.4. Most Frequent Herbs in Citations Related to Chronic Cough

Herb Name	Scientific Name	No. of Citations (*n*)
Sheng jiang 生姜	*Zingiber officinale* (Willd.) Rosc.	133
Feng mi 蜂蜜	Honey	122
Gan cao 甘草	*Glycyrrhizae spp.*	107
Kuan dong hua 款冬花	*Tussilago farfara* L.	88
Xing ren 杏仁	*Prunus armeniaca* L.	82
Ren shen 人参	*Panax ginseng* C. A. Mey.	75
Zi wan 紫菀	*Aster tataricus* L.f.	64
Sang gen bai pi 桑根白皮/ *Sang bai pi* 桑白皮	*Morus alba* L.	61
Wu wei zi 五味子	*Chisandra chinensis* (Turcz.) Baill.	60
Bei mu 贝母	*Fritillaria cirrhosa* D. Don	47
Chen pi 陈皮	*Citrus tangerina* Hort.et Tanaka and *Citrus erythrosa* Tanaka	46
Ban xia 半夏	*Pinellia ternata* (Thunb.) Breit.	41
Jie geng 桔梗	*Platycodon grandiflorum* (Jacq.) A.DC.	40
E jiao 阿胶	*Equue asinus* L.	36
Da zao 大枣	*Ziziphus jujuba* Mill. Var. inermis (Bge.) Rehd.	35
Rou gui 肉桂	*Cinnamomum cassia* Presl	33
Fu ling 茯苓	*Poria cocos* (Schw.) Wolf	30
Wu mei 乌梅	*Prunus mume* (Sieb.) Sieb. and Zucc.	27
Xi xin 细辛	*Asarum heterotropoides* F. Schm. var. mandshuricum (Maxim) Kitag.	25
Ying su ke 罂粟壳	*Papaver somniferum* L.	25

The use of some herbs/ingredients may be restricted in some countries. For example, herbs such as *xi xin* 细辛 and *ying su ke* 罂粟壳 can be toxic. Readers are advised to comply with relevant regulations.

- Constrain the Lung to suppress cough such as *wu mei* 乌梅, *wu wei zi* 五味子 and *ying su ke* 罂粟壳;
- Warm the Lung, dissipate cold and resolve cough, such as *sheng jiang* 生姜 and *xi xin* 细辛;
- Clear heat and resolve phlegm, such as *bei mu* 贝母 and *sang bai pi* 桑白皮;

- Direct *qi* downward to suppress cough, such as *kuan dong hua* 款冬花, *zi wan* 紫菀, and *xing ren* 杏仁;
- Dry dampness to resolve phlegm, such as *chen pi* 陈皮 and *ban xia* 半夏.

Three most frequently mentioned ingredients, *sheng jiang* 生姜 (*n* = 133), *feng mi* 蜂蜜 (*n* = 122) and *gan cao* 甘草 (*n* = 107) were obtained from more than 100 citations. *Sheng jiang* 生姜 has the therapeutic function of releasing the exterior, dissipating cold, warming the Lung and suppressing cough.[9] It has been, and still is, widely used for treating chronic cough due to cold in the Lungs. It should be noted that in many citations, *sheng jiang* 生姜 was used as an assistant ingredient within the formula and may not be individually identified as a herb for cough, but as an assistant to the other herbs. In one citation from *Ji Yang Gang Mu* 济阳纲目 (c. 1626), it was stated that '*Gu er mu san* 古二母散 could be used for treating acute or chronic cough, and asthma with sputum … It should be taken before sleep by chewing several pieces of *sheng jiang* 生姜, and with *sheng jiang* 生姜 decoction' (古二母散 治远年近日诸般咳嗽, 兼治痰喘…每服一字, 姜三片临卧细嚼, 姜汤下…).

Feng mi 蜂蜜 (honey), which moistens the Lung and suppresses cough, was also mentioned as an assistant ingredient in the included citations. It was often used as an excipient when preparing/producing the CHMs into pill form, such as 'add *Feng mi* 蜂蜜, mix the herbs and rub them to pills' (炼蜜和丸). In *Ben Cao Gang Mu* 本草纲目 (c.1578), *feng mi* 蜂蜜 was mentioned to have the function of harmonising the herbs and having similar function to *gan cao* 甘草. The clinical function of suppressing cough and harmonising other herbs in the formula could be an explanation of *feng mi's* popularity in classical literature.

Gan cao 甘草 is widely used in formulation in CHM to harmonise other herbs as an assisting ingredient, which may contribute to its high frequency in classical literature. *Gan cao* 甘草 also has the function of tonifying Spleen *qi* and resolving phlegm to suppress cough. It is beneficial for treating chronic cough generated by Spleen and Lung *qi* deficiency, and phlegm accumulating in Spleen and Lung. For example, in *Wei Sheng Jian Yi Fang* 卫生简易方 (c. 1410), *gan cao* 甘草 was selected for treating chronic cough due to phlegm in the Lungs, runny nose, coughing up sputum and feeling joint discomfort ('治肺痰久嗽, 涕唾多, 骨节烦闷寒热, 用甘草炙为末'). Recent experimental studies also suggest constituents isolated from *gan cao* 甘草 have potent antitussive, antispasmodic and anti-inflammatory functions (see Chapter 6).

Kuan dong hua 款冬花, the fourth most frequently cited herb, moistens the Lungs to direct *qi* downward, resolving phlegm and suppressing cough. It was widely used in cough-suppressing formulas historically. In *Ben Cao Zheng Yi* 本草正义 (c. 1920), the author pointed out that *kuan dong hua* 款冬花 can be used for managing various lung diseases. It has the function to diffuse the Lung and resolve *qi* stagnation, relieve Lung *qi* ascending counterflow and asthma, especially beneficial for managing cough ('款冬花主肺病, 能开泄郁结, 定逆止喘, 专主咳嗽').

Xing ren 杏仁, mentioned in 82 citations, was the fifth most commonly used herb. Similar to *kuan dong hua* 款冬花, *xing ren* 杏仁 functions to direct *qi* downward and suppress cough, clear phlegm and moisten the Lung, Spleen and Stomach (*Dian Nan Ben Cao* 滇南本草, c.1436, 杏仁, 止咳嗽, 消痰润肺, 润肠胃).

It should also be noted that two toxic ingredients, *xi xin* 细辛 and *ying su ke* 罂粟壳, were identified in the most frequently reported herbs in the citation pool, which are restricted in some countries. *Xi xin* 细辛 (*Asarum heterotropoides* F. Schm. var. mandshuricum (Maxim) Kitag.), is a herb traditionally used for warming the Lung meridian and resolving fluid retention. In recent years, the safety concern of *xi xin* 细辛 has arisen due to it containing aristolochic acids which may lead to renal failure.[10] In clinical practice, *xi xin* 细辛 could be replaced with other herbs carrying similar functions, such as *fang feng* paired with *gui zhi*, or *gan jiang* paired with *ban xia*.[9]

Ying su ke 罂粟壳 (*Papaver somniferum* L.), the capsule shell of the poppy seed, carries the function of constraining the Lung to suppress cough. The compounds morphine, codeine and alkaloids in *ying su ke* 罂粟壳 have strong antitussive therapeutic effects, but they may also induce serious side effects such as breathing difficulties and addiction when inappropriately used. This herb has been widely restricted globally.[11]

Table 3.5.   Most Frequent Single Herb Formulas for Chronic Cough

Herb Name	Scientific Name	Number of Citations (*n*)
Bai bu 百部	*Stemona sessilifolia* (Miq.) Miq.	10
Kuan dong hua 款冬花	*Tussilago farfara* L.	5
Mu fu rong ye 木芙蓉叶	*Hibiscus mutabilis* L.	3

Single Herb Formulas in Citations Related to Chronic Cough

Twenty herbs were identified as 'single herb formula' and were analysed as a subset of the data. Three herbs, *bai bu* 百部, *kuan dong hua* 款冬花 and *mu fu rong ye* 木芙蓉叶, were identified in multiple citations (Table 3.5).

Bai bu 百部 was the most frequently mentioned single herb formula. The earliest mention was from the book *Wai Tai Mi Yao* 外台秘要 (c. 752). The author, Wang Tao, mentioned a formula and the preparation method to treat '30-year chronic cough'. It says to mash the root of *bai bu* 百部 and get the juice, then boil the juice and concentrate it as a sugar. *Bai bu* 百部 is used to moisten the Lung and direct *qi* downward to suppress cough, which is beneficial for relieving chronic cough related to the Lung dryness and *qi* deficiency. The herb *kuan dong hua* 款冬花 also moistens the Lung and suppresses coughing while *mu fu rong ye* 木芙蓉叶 clears Lung heat and cools the Blood.

Acupuncture and Related Therapies

A total of 29 citations describing acupuncture and related therapies met the inclusion criteria and were included for analysis. The eligible citations were identified from 20 books. *Bian Que Xin Shu* 扁鹊新书 (c. 1146) (*n* = 3) and *Zhen Jiu Feng Yuan* 针灸逢源 (c. 1882) (*n* = 3) were the only two books that yielded more than one citation.

Frequency of Treatment Citations by Dynasty

The included citations were identified from the books published from the Song and Jin dynasties to the Qing dynasty (Table 3.6).

Table 3.6. Dynastic Distribution of Treatment Citations

Dynasty	No. of Treatment Citations
Song and Jin dynasties (961–1271)	6
Ming dynasty (1369–1644)	9
Qing dynasty (1645–1911)	14
Total	29

Consistent with the CHM citations, books published during the Ming dynasty (c. 1369–1644) and the Qing dynasty (c. 1645–1911) contributed the largest number ($n = 23$, 79%).

The earliest citation was obtained from the book *Sheng Ji Zong Lu* 圣济总录 (c. 1117), which was identified by the search term *jiu ke* 久咳. Two acupuncture points, TE10 *Tianjing* 天井 and TE6 *Zhigou* 支沟, were recommended to manage chronic cough with fullness and oedema. The most recent citation was identified from *Jiu Fa Mi Chuan* 灸法秘传 (c. 1883) by the search term *jiu sou* 久嗽. It mentioned that chronic cough with overexertion or heat symptoms could be treated by moxibustion on BL13 *Feishu* 肺俞.

Treatment with Acupuncture and Related Therapies

Of the included 29 acupuncture and related therapies citations, 19 described moxibustion for managing chronic cough (65.5%), while eight mentioned acupuncture as treatment and two recommended combination of these two therapies (Table 3.7). The results suggested that moxibustion might be a popular therapy for managing chronic cough in dynastic China. Acupuncture points were extracted from the included citations for further analysis.

Table 3.7. Acupuncture Treatments in Citations Related to Chronic Cough

Acupuncture Treatment	No. of Citations (n)
Acupuncture	8
Acupuncture and moxibustion	2
Moxibustion	19

Most Frequent Acupuncture Points

A total of 25 acupuncture points were obtained from the included citations. Twelve acupuncture points were found in multiple citations (Table 3.8). The acupoint BL13 *Feishu* 肺俞 was the most cited acupuncture point in the citations (*n* = 9). It is a back-shu point of the Lung and stimulating this point can tonify Lung *qi* and *yin*, clear deficient heat from the Lung, and release the exterior. Six of the included citations recommend moxibustion therapy on this point for managing chronic cough, suggesting its importance in treating chronic cough with Lung *qi* and *yin* deficiency syndrome. Many of the most frequently cited acupuncture points are located on the neck and chest region, which might indicate the selection of these adjacent points were according to the local therapeutic effect of acupuncture points.

A cluster of acupuncture points located on the abdomen area (CV10 *Xiawan* 下脘 and CV4 *Guanyuan* 关元) or from the Stomach meridian (ST36 *Zusanli* 足三里) were also frequently mentioned in the classical literature for chronic cough. These points can tonify Spleen and Stomach *qi*, dispel dampness and resolve phlegm.

Table 3.8.   Most Frequent Acupuncture Points

Acupuncture Point	No. of Citations (*n*)
BL13 *Feishu* 肺俞	9
EX-HN10 *Juquan* 聚泉	6
BL43 *Gaohuanshu* 膏肓俞	4
GV10 *Lingtai* 灵台	3
ST18 *Rugen* 乳根	3
BL12 *Fengmen* 风门	2
CV10 *Xiawan* 下脘	2
CV17 *Danzhong* 膻中	2
CV4 *Guanyuan* 关元	2
ST12 *Quepen* 缺盆	2
ST36 *Zusanli* 足三里	2
TE10 *Tianjing* 天井	2

Stimulating these points could be beneficial for chronic cough related to disfunction of the Spleen and Stomach.

Other Chinese Medicine Therapies

A total of 52 citations described other CM therapies for managing chronic cough. The majority introduced herbal smoke inhaling therapy (*n* = 46). Two citations recommended diet therapy, or herb scrubbing/washing therapy, and one citation mentioned bloodletting therapy or *huo jiao fa* 火角法 for chronic cough, but no details related to this treatment were described (Table 3.9). All these therapies, excluding diet therapy, are quite unconventional compared to modern clinical practice. However, they are still described for reader interest.

The earliest citation of herbal smoke inhaling therapy was from the book *Zhou Hou Bei Ji Fang* 肘后备急方 published in the Dongjin dynasty (c. AD 363). The author, Ge Hong, detailed the preparation of equipment for inhaling therapy using an iron griddle and bamboo. The patient should inhale the *kuan dong hua* 款冬花 smoke from the heated equipment for five days, after which the patient will recover (每旦取款冬花如鸡子许, 少蜜拌花使润, 纳一升铁铛中, 又用一瓦碗钻一孔, 孔内安一小竹筒, 笔管亦得, 其筒稍长, 作碗铛相合, 及撞筒处, 皆面泥之, 勿令漏气, 铛下着炭, 少时款冬烟自从筒出. 则口含筒, 吸取烟咽之. 如胸中少闷, 须举头, 即将指头捻筒头, 勿使漏烟气,

Table 3.9.　Other Chinese Medicine Therapies for Chronic Cough

Other Chinese Medicine Treatment Methods	No. of Citations (*n*)
Herbal smoke inhaling therapy	46
Diet therapy	2
Herbs scrubbing/washing	2
Bloodletting	1
Huo jiao fa 火角法 (no details specified)	1
Total	52

吸烟使尽止. 凡如是五日一为之,　待至六日,　则饱食羊肉馎饦一顿, 永瘥).

In the book *Yi Xue Yuan Li* 医学原理 (c. 1644), herbal smoke inhaling therapy was used in combination with moxibustion: 'Grind *e guan shi* 鹅管石, *xiong huang* 雄黄, *yu jin* 郁金, and *kuan dong hua* 款冬花 together to powder. Place one piece of *sheng jiang* 生姜 on the patient's tongue. Mix the powder with *ai ye* 艾叶 and burn the mixture, then ask the patient to inhale the herbal smoke.' (如风入肺久嗽者, 用鹅管石, 雄黄, 郁金, 款冬花为末, 以生姜一片置舌上, 以艾拌药末于姜上灸之, 吸烟入喉). *Kuan dong hua* 款冬花 was the most frequently used herb for smoke inhaling therapy; it moistens the Lungs, resolves phlegm and suppresses cough. Herbal smoke inhaling therapy is unconventional in contemporary CM guidelines and textbooks, although it was mentioned in various classical literature.

Classical Literature in Perspective

Chronic cough was a common condition that was described in many classical literature citations. In many citations, chronic cough wasn't diagnosed with strict criteria; rather, the symptoms were described. The aetiology and pathogenesis of chronic cough have been discussed in depth in classical literature. Consistent with contemporary CM literature, the understanding of chronic cough included citations that detailed dysfunction of different *zang* and *fu*, and that could all lead to chronic cough. Fire, heat and dryness were the most frequently mentioned pathogens in the included citations that caused disordered diffusion of Lung *qi* manifesting as chronic cough.

Most of the identified citations were found in books published in the Ming dynasty (c. 1369–1644) and the Qing dynasty (c. 1645–1911). The first citation that mentioned treatment of chronic cough was obtained from the *Zhou Hou Bei Ji Fang* 肘后备急方 (c. 363 AD). *E jiao san* 阿胶散 was the most frequently described formula to treat chronic cough, which carries the clinical functions of tonifying *qi* and *yin*, supressing cough and resolving phlegm. The key clinical functions of the most frequently reported formulas and herbs were similar, including suppressing cough and resolving phlegm.

The evidence of acupuncture and related therapies for chronic cough was limited. Moxibustion was found to be a popular therapy for chronic cough, with BL13 *Feishu* 肺俞 the most frequently mentioned acupuncture point. In contemporary CM practice, manual acupuncture and moxibustion on BL13 *Feishu* 肺俞 is recommended by the clinical guidelines. This suggests that the evidence from the classical literature continues to influence current CM practice.

The included citations also introduced several other CM therapies for chronic cough, including herbal smoke inhaling therapy, diet therapy, herb scrubbing/washing therapy and bloodletting therapy. Although these therapies are not conventionally used in contemporary CM practice, they enrich the understanding of treatment methods for chronic cough in dynastic China.

References

1. Needham J, Lu G, Sivin N. (2000) *Science and Civilisation in China. Volume 5, Part VI: Medicine.* Cambridge University Press, UK.
2. Hu R, ed. (2000) *Encyclopedia of Traditional Chinese Medicine.* Hunan Electronic and Audio-Visual Publishing House, Changsha.
3. May B, Lu C, Xue CC. (2012) Collections of traditional Chinese medical litearture as resources for systematic searches. *J Altern Complement Med* **18(12):** 1101–1107.
4. May B, Lu Y, Lu C, *et al.* (2013) Systematic assessment of the representativeness of published collections of the traditional literature on Chinese medicine. *J Altern Complement Med* **19(5):** 403–409.
5. 中华中医药学会内科分会肺系病专业委员会, 咳嗽中医诊疗专家共识意见. (2011) 中医杂志 **52(10):** 896–899.
6. 周仲英. (2003) 中医内科学. 北京: 中国中医药出版社.
7. 朱文锋. (1999) 国家标准应用·中医内科疾病诊疗常规. 湖南: 湖南科学技术出版社.
8. 王永炎, 鲁兆麟. (1999) 中医内科学. 北京: 人民卫生出版社.
9. 唐德才, 吴庆光. (2017) 中药学. 北京: 人民卫生出版社.

10. Kumar V, Poonam, Pradad AK, *et al.* (2003) Naturally occurring aristol-actams, aristolochic acids and dioxoaporphines and their biological activities. *Nat Prod Rep* **20(6):** 565–583.
11. Hao DC, Gu XJ, Xiao PG. (2015) Chapter 6: Phytochemical and biological research of Papaver pharmaceutical resources. In: Hao DC, Gu XJ, Xiao PG (eds), *Medicinal Plants.* Woodhead Publishing, UK, pp. 217–251.

4

Methods for Evaluating Clinical Evidence

OVERVIEW

This chapter describes the methods used to identify and evaluate a range of Chinese medicine interventions for chronic cough in clinical studies. Studies identified through a comprehensive search were assessed against eligibility criteria. A review of the methodological quality of the studies was undertaken using standardised methods. Results from included studies were evaluated to provide an estimate of the effects of a range of Chinese medicine therapies.

Introduction

The use of Chinese medicine (CM) for chronic cough, including the subtypes of cough variant asthma (CVA), upper airways cough syndrome (UACS) and gastro-oesophageal reflux disease (GORD) has been well described in contemporary and classical CM literature. Several systematic reviews have been conducted to evaluate the efficacy and safety of CM treatment for chronic cough. This has included seven reviews of Chinese herbal medicines (CHMs). Systematic reviews have been summarised in the relevant chapters.

This chapter includes the methods of examining the CM interventions for chronic cough in clinical studies. Efficacy and safety will be examined in controlled clinical trials. Interventions have been categorised as follows: CHM (Chapter 5) and acupuncture and related therapies (Chapter 7).

References to clinical trials were obtained and assessed by an expert group. Randomised controlled trials (RCTs), non-randomised controlled clinical trials (CCTs) and non-controlled studies were evaluated in detail. Controlled trials were evaluated using the same approach as RCTs, and have been described separately. Evidence from non-controlled studies is more difficult to evaluate; therefore the approach was taken to describe the characteristics of the study, details of the intervention and any adverse events. References to included studies are indicated by a letter followed by a number. Studies of CHM are indicated by an 'H' e.g. H1, studies of acupuncture and related therapies indicated by an 'A' e.g. A1.

Search Strategy

Evidence was searched in English- and Chinese-language databases and the methods followed the Cochrane Handbook of Systematic Reviews.[1] English-language databases included PubMed, Excerpta Medica Database (Embase), Cumulative Index of Nursing and Allied Health Literature (CINAHL), Cochrane Central Register of Controlled Trials (CENTRAL) including the Cochrane Library, and Allied and Complementary Medicine Database (AMED); Chinese-language databases included China BioMedical Literature (CBM), China National Knowledge Infrastructure (CNKI), Chongqing VIP (CQVIP) and Wanfang. Databases were searched from inception to May 2018. No restrictions were applied. Search terms were mapped to controlled vocabulary (where applicable) in addition to being searched as keywords.

To conduct a comprehensive search of the literature, searches were run according to the study design (reviews, controlled trials and non-controlled studies). This was done for each of the three intervention types (CHM, acupuncture and related therapies, and other CM therapies) resulting in nine searches in each of the nine databases:

1. CHM reviews;
2. CHM controlled trials (randomised and non-randomised);
3. CHM non-controlled studies;
4. Acupuncture and related therapies — reviews;
5. Acupuncture and related therapies — controlled trials (randomised and non-randomised);
6. Acupuncture and related therapies — non-controlled studies;

7. Other CM therapies — reviews;
8. Other CM therapies — controlled trials (randomised and non-randomised);
9. Other CM therapies — non-controlled studies.

Studies of combination CM therapies were identified through the above searches. In addition to electronic databases, reference lists of systematic reviews and included studies were searched for additional publications. Clinical trials registries were searched to identify clinical trials which were ongoing or completed, and where required, trial investigators were contacted to obtain data. Trial investigators were contacted by email or telephone and were followed up after two weeks if no reply was received. Where no response was received after one month, any unknown information was marked as not available. The searched trial registries included the Australian New Zealand Clinical Trial Registry (ANZCTR), the Chinese Clinical Trial Registry (ChiCTR), the European Union Clinical Trials Register (EU-CTR) and the United States of America National Institutes of Health register (ClinicalTrials.gov).

Inclusion Criteria

- Study type: Controlled prospective studies with or without randomisation, and uncontrolled studies (cohort, case series and case studies);
- Participants: Aged over 18 years old with the main complaint of cough for eight weeks or more. Cough subtypes included CVA, UACS or GORD diagnosed by relevant clinical practice guidelines, such as the American College of Chest Physicians (ACCP) diagnosis and management of cough,[2] the European Respiratory Society (ERS) diagnosis and management of chronic cough[3] or the Chinese national guidelines on diagnosis and management of cough;[4]
- Interventions: Chinese herbal medicine, acupuncture and related therapies, or other CM therapies, alone or in combination with other CM therapies or with pharmacotherapy/routine care. Studies combining CM therapies with pharmacotherapy/routine care required the use of the same pharmacotherapy/routine care in both the intervention and comparator groups;

- Comparators: Placebo, pharmacotherapies or other routine care therapies that are recommended in clinical practice guidelines;
- Outcome measures: Studies reported at least one of the pre-specified outcome measures (Table 4.1).

Table 4.1.   Pre-specified Outcomes

Outcome Measures	Scoring
Leicester Cough Questionnaire (LCQ)[5]	19 items; higher scores indicate less symptoms
Cough-Specific Quality-of-Life Questionnaire (CQLQ)[6]	28 items; higher scores indicate less symptoms
Cough symptom score	Scoring varies based on the measure used; 0–10 visual analogue scale is common
Coughing reflex sensitivity	Varies based on the measure used
Cough symptom improvement (including cough diary)	Varies based on the provocation tests used; 0–10 visual analogue scale is common
Lung function (cough variant asthma [CVA] subgroup)	• Forced expiratory volume in one second (FEV_1) • Forced vital capacity (FVC) • Peak expiratory flow
Fractional exhaled nitric oxide (FeNO) (CVA subgroup)	• Higher scores indicate more severe disease
Eosinophil counts (CVA subgroup)	• Blood eosinophil count; higher scores indicate more severe disease • Induced sputum eosinophil cationic protein (ECP); higher scores indicate more severe disease
Reflux Disease Questionnaire (GORD subgroup)	12 items; higher scores indicate more symptoms

Effective rate[7–9]	• Number of people with improved symptoms and signs
	• Curative effect:
	  ○ Clinically controlled
	  ○ Markedly effective
	  ○ Effective
	  ○ Ineffective
	
	Curative effect categories were combined for analysis into effective or ineffective

Adverse events	Number and type of adverse events

Exclusion Criteria

- Study type: Epidemiological studies, studies that compared CM therapy to other CM therapies, and duplicated studies reporting the same results;
- Participants: Acute cough, or sub-acute cough lasting less than 8 weeks, drug-induced cough (e.g. from Angiotensin-converting enzyme [ACE] inhibitors), chemical/occupational-induced cough, cardiac cough (e.g. congestive heart failure), psychological cough (e.g. stress-induced, depression), neoplastic cough (e.g. lung cancer), and idiopathic cough. Trials of other respiratory disorders where chronic cough is not the key disorder such as asthma or chronic obstructive pulmonary disease;
- Intervention: Chinese medicine interventions not commonly practiced worldwide and CM intra venous interventions;
- Comparators: Control not routinely recommended for chronic cough in international clinical practice guidelines or no treatment control. Control therapies that included any type of CM therapies. Integrative medicine studies that used different therapies in the intervention groups compared to the control group.

Outcomes

Pre-specified outcomes of effect included known measures in chronic cough research including cough questionnaires, cough sensitivity, quality of life, and adverse events. The outcomes and measurements are specified in Table 4.1.

Risk of Bias Assessment

Risk of bias was assessed for randomised controlled trials using the Cochrane Collaboration's tool.[1] In clinical trials, bias can be categorised as selection bias, performance bias, detection bias, attrition bias and reporting bias. Each domain is assessed to determine whether the bias is at 'low', 'high' or 'unclear' risk. 'Low' risk of bias indicates that bias is unlikely, 'high' risk indicates plausible bias that seriously weakens confidence in the results and 'unclear' bias indicates lack of information or uncertainty over potential bias, thus raising some doubt about the results. Risk of bias assessment was verified by two people and disagreement was resolved by discussion or consultation with a third person.

Risk of bias is categorised using the following six domains:

- Sequence generation: The method used to generate the allocation sequence is given in sufficient detail to allow an assessment of whether it should produce comparable groups. 'Low' risk of bias refers to a random number table or computer random generator. 'High' risk of bias includes studies that describe a non-random sequence generation such as odd or even date of birth or date of admission;
- Allocation concealment: The method used to conceal the allocation sequence is given in enough detail to determine whether intervention allocations could have been foreseen before or during enrolment. 'Low' risk of bias includes central randomisation or sealed envelopes and 'high' risk of bias includes open random sequence;
- Blinding of participants and personnel: Measures used to describe if the study participants and personnel are blind to the intervention received. In addition, information relating to whether the blinding was effective is also assessed. Studies that ensure blinding of participants and personnel are at 'low' risk of bias. If the study is not blind or incompletely blind, it is at 'high' risk of bias;
- Blinding of outcome assessors: Measures used to describe if the outcome assessors are blind to knowledge of which intervention a participant received. In addition, information relating to whether the blinding was effective is also assessed. Studies that ensure blinding of outcome assessors are at 'low' risk of bias. If the study is not blind or incompletely blind, it is at 'high' risk of bias;
- Incomplete outcome data: Completeness of outcome data for each main outcome, including drop-outs, exclusions from the analysis

with numbers missing in each group and reasons for drop-out or exclusions. Studies with 'low' risk of bias would include all outcome data or if there is missing data it is unlikely to relate to the true outcome or is balanced between groups. Studies at 'high' risk of bias would have unexplained missing data;

- Selective reporting: The study protocol is available and the pre-specified outcomes are included in the report. Studies with a published protocol and which include all pre-specified outcomes in their report would be at 'low' risk of bias. Studies at 'high' risk of bias would not include all pre-specified outcomes or the outcome data may be reported incompletely.

Statistical Analyses

The results of the different subtypes of chronic cough, CVA, UACS and GORD are reported separately. Frequency of CM syndromes, CHM formulas, herbs and acupuncture points reported in the included studies are presented using descriptive statistics. Chinese medicine syndromes reported in two or more studies were presented. The ten most frequently reported CHM formulas and 20 most frequently reported herbs are presented (if used in at least two studies), although for CHM formulas, this was not always possible. The frequently used acupuncture points are also presented. Where data were limited, reports of single CM syndromes or acupuncture points were provided as a guide for the reader.

Definitions of statistical tests and results are described in the glossary. Dichotomous data are reported as a risk ratio (RR) with 95% confidence intervals (CI) and continuous data are reported as mean difference (MD) or standardised mean difference (SMD) with 95% CI. For dichotomous data, when the RR is greater than one and the upper and lower values of the 95% CI are both greater than one, this indicates we can be 95% certain that there is a difference between the groups and that the true effect lies within these CIs. The same is true for values less than one. In such cases, we say there is a 'significant difference' between the groups. For continuous data, when the MD is greater than zero and both the upper and lower values of the 95% CI are greater than zero, we say there is a 'significant difference' between the groups. The same is true on the negative side of the scale.[1] For all analyses, RR or MD and 95% CI were reported, together with a formal test for heterogeneity using the I^2 statistic. An I^2 score greater than 50% was considered to indicate substantial heterogeneity.[1] Sensitivity analyses were undertaken to explore potential sources of heterogeneity, based on 'low' risk of bias for one of the risk of bias domains, sequence generation. Where possible and appropriate, planned subgroup analyses included duration of treatment, CM syndromes, CM formula and comparator type. Available case analysis with a random effects model was used in all analyses. The random effects model was used to take into account the clinical heterogeneity likely to be encountered within, and between, included studies and the variation in treatment effects between included studies.

Assessment Using Grading of Recommendations Assessment, Development and Evaluation

The Grading of Recommendations Assessment, Development and Evaluation (GRADE) approach was used.[10–11] The GRADE approach summarises and rates the certainty of evidence in systematic reviews using a structured process for presenting evidence summaries. The results are presented in summary of findings tables. The results provide an important overview for chronic cough outcomes.

A panel of experts was established to evaluate the certainty of evidence. The panel included the systematic review team, CM practitioners, integrative medicine experts, research methodologists and conventional medicine physicians. The experts were asked to rate the clinical importance of key interventions from CHM, acupuncture therapies and other CM therapies, as well as comparators and outcomes. Results were collated and based on the rating scores and subsequent discussion, and a consensus on the content for the summary of findings tables was achieved.

The certainty of evidence for each outcome was rated according to five factors outlined in the GRADE approach. The quality of evidence may be rated based on the following:

- Limitations in study design (risk of bias);
- Inconsistency of results (unexplained heterogeneity);
- Indirectness of evidence (interventions, populations and outcomes important to the patients with the condition);
- Imprecision (uncertainty about the results);
- Publication bias (selective publication of studies).

These five factors are additive, and a reduction in more than one factor will reduce the certainty of the evidence for that outcome.

Treatment recommendations can also be assessed using the GRADE approach but due to the diverse nature of CM practice, treatment recommendations were not included with the summary of findings. Therefore, the reader should interpret the evidence with reference to the local practice environment. It should also be noted that the GRADE approach requires judgments about the quality of evidence and some subjective assessment. However, the experience of the panel members suggests the judgments are reliable and transparent representations of the quality of evidence.

The GRADE levels of evidence are grouped into four categories:

1. 'High' certainty evidence: We are very confident that the true effect lies close to that of the estimate of the effect;
2. 'Moderate' certainty evidence: We are moderately confident in the effect estimate. The true effect is likely to be close to the estimate of the effect, but there is a possibility that it is substantially different;
3. 'Low' certainty evidence: Our confidence in the effect estimate is limited. The true effect may be substantially different from the estimate of the effect;
4. 'Very low' certainty evidence: We have very little confidence in the effect estimate. The true effect is likely to be substantially different from the estimate of effect.

References

1. Higgins J, Green S, eds. (2011) *Cochrane Handbook for Systematic Reviews of Interventions Version 5.1.0.* The Cochrane Collaboration. Available from: http://www.cochrane-handbook.org.
2. Irwin RS, Baumann MH, Bolser DC, *et al.* (2006) Diagnosis and management of cough executive summary: ACCP evidence-based clinical practice guidelines. *Chest* **129(Suppl 1):** S1–S23.
3. Morice AH, Fontana GA, Sovijarvi AR, *et al.* (2004) The diagnosis and management of chronic cough. *Eur Respir J* **24(3):** 481–492.
4. Asthma Workgroup of Chinese Society of Respiratory Diseases, Chinese Medicine Association. (2011) The Chinese national guidelines on diagnosis and management of cough. *Chin Med J* **124:** 3207–3219.
5. Birring SS, Prudon B, Carr AJ, *et al.* (2003) Development of a symptom-specific health status measure for patients with chronic cough: Leicester Cough Questionnaire (LCQ). *Thorax* **58(4):** 339–343.
6. French CT, Irwin RS, Fletcher KE, Adams TM. (2002) Evaluation of a cough-specific quality-of-life questionnaire. *Chest* **121(4):** 1123–1131.
7. Clinical guidelines of new drugs of traditional Chinese medicine (2002) [In Chinese: 2002版, 中药新药临床指导原则, — 性支气管炎].
8. Criteria of diagnosis and therapeutic effect of internal medicine diseases and syndromes in traditional Chinese medicine (2016) [In Chinese: 中医内科病证诊断疗效标准].
9. Routine methods of diagnosis and treatment of common diseases in department of TCM (2013) [In Chinese: 中医科常见病诊疗常规].
10. Schunemann H, Brozek J, Guyatt G, Oxman A, eds. (2013) *GRADE Handbook for Grading Quality of Evidence and Strength of Recommendations.* The GRADE Working Group. Available from: http://www.guidelinedevelopment.org/handbook/.
11. Schunemann HJ, Higgins JPT, Vist GE, *et al.* Chapter 14: Completing 'summary of findings' tables and grading the certainty of the evidence. In: Higgins JPT, Thomas J, Chandler J, *et al.*, eds. (2019) *Cochrane Handbook for Systematic Reviews of Interventions Version 6.0* (updated July 2019). Available from: http://www.training.cochrane.org/handbook/.

5

Clinical Evidence for Chinese Herbal Medicine

OVERVIEW

This chapter provides an overview of the clinical evidence of Chinese herbal medicine in the management of chronic cough, including cough subtypes of cough variant asthma, upper airways cough syndrome and gastro-oesophageal reflux disease-related cough. Randomised controlled trials, non-randomised controlled clinical trials and non-controlled studies were identified by searching nine English and Chinese electronic medical databases. Systematic reviews and descriptive analyses were used to evaluate the efficacy and safety of the Chinese herbal medicines for chronic cough. The results will help to guide readers to better understand the overall evidence of CHM in the treatment of chronic cough.

Introduction

Chinese herbal medicine (CHM) is guided by the theory of traditional Chinese medicine (CM) to collect, process, prepare and administer herbal medicines for disease prevention and treatment. Chinese herbal medicine includes botanicals (roots, stems, leaves and fruits), animal products (viscera, skin, bones and organs) and mineral medicines, used in combinations called formula. The administration types of CHM also vary, and include decoctions, liquid extracts, ointments, pills, capsules and powders.

Chronic cough is defined as cough lasting longer than eight weeks, with cough as the primary or sole symptom (see Chapter 1).

Chronic cough refers to cough variant asthma (CVA), upper airway cough syndrome (UACS) and gastro-oesophageal reflux disease-related cough (GORD-C). Chinese herbal medicine for chronic cough has been assessed in numerous clinical trials. Systematic reviews and descriptive analysis were performed to determine the efficacy and safety of CHM for chronic cough in adults.

Previous Systematic Reviews

Systematic reviews have been published on CHM for chronic cough. They evaluate the efficacy of CHM alone or in combination with conventional medicines such as inhaled corticosteroids (ICS), bronchodilators, and leukotriene receptor antagonists. All reviews evaluated CVA, except for one that evaluated people with UACS. There were no systematic reviews of GORD-C.

Two systematic reviews have evaluated the efficacy of *Su huang zhi ke jiao nang* 苏黄止咳胶囊 for CVA.[1–2] Results from both reviews showed that *Su huang zhi ke jiao nang* was superior to pharmacotherapies in terms of improved clinical efficacy, and one review reported decreased occurrence of adverse events.[1] Nevertheless, the authors indicated that more large-scale, high-quality randomised controlled trials (RCTs) are needed to confirm their results.

Wu *et al.* (2015) and Dai *et al.* (2017) assessed the efficacy and safety of all types of CHM for CVA.[3–4] The pooled results from one review of 17 RCTs showed that CHM alone was superior to pharmacotherapies and reduced cough symptoms, but there was no difference in terms of total effective rate and airway hyper-reactivity.[3] The other review included 21 studies and showed CHM was superior to ICS plus bronchodilator, and that total effective rate was increased and airway sensitivity and occurrence of cough reduced.[4] However, in terms of lung function, blood eosinophils, total immunoglobulin E (IgE) and inflammatory factors, there was no difference between CHM and ICS/bronchodilator groups. The authors commented that although the overall result was positive, it was premature to confirm the efficacy of CHM for CVA due to the lack of high-quality studies.

In 2016, Chen *et al.* evaluated the efficacy and safety of *Huang qi xi xin tang* 黄芪细辛汤 for CVA by conducting a systematic review and meta-analysis.[5] Three RCTs, including 192 participants, were included. The pooled results showed *Huang qi xi xin tang* was superior to pharmacotherapies at decreasing airway reaction, but there was no difference in terms of total effective rate. No adverse reactions were reported by participants taking *Huang qi xi xin tang*. The shortcoming of the review was that the number of studies was small and the quality was 'low'.

In 2017, Pan *et al.* reported evidence of *Gui zhi jia hou po xing zi tang* 桂枝加厚朴杏子汤 for CVA.[6] Six RCTs, including 1,142 participants, were included. The primary outcome measures were total effective rate and safety. Results indicated that *Gui zhi jia xing zi tang* alone or combined with conventional medicine could increase clinical efficacy. As for safety, *Gui zhi jia xing zi tang* had fewer adverse events than conventional medicine. Nevertheless, the authors indicated that further high-quality studies with better methodology should be conducted because the number of studies was small, and the quality of studies was 'low.'

Wu *et al.* (2017) reported the efficacy and safety of *Jia wei xiao chai hu tang* 加味小柴胡汤 for CVA.[7] The systematic review included 11 studies with 918 participants and showed that *Jia wei xiao chai hu tang* was superior to pharmacotherapies and improved total effective rate and decreased occurrence of cough. Nevertheless, this conclusion still needs to be validated by high-quality, double-blinded RCTs.

For UACS, a systematic review of 16 RCTs was published by Jiang *et al.* in 2016.[8] It indicated that total effective rate, cough symptom scores, symptoms of cough and postnasal drip were improved after CHM treatment alone, or combined with pharmacotherapies, compared to placebo or pharmacotherapies alone. One systematic review assessed CHM for non-acute bronchial asthma complicated by gastro-oesophageal reflux.[9] Six RCTs were included involving 304 patients. Chinese herbal medicine was used alone or combined with anti-inflammatory drugs, bronchodilators and drugs to promote gastric peristalsis and inhibit gastric acid production for gastro-oesophageal reflux. Results favoured the CHM treatments in terms of clinical efficacy, symptom scores, pulmonary function values and adverse events. However, similar to the systematic reviews of CVA and UACS, there was a small number of studies with few participants, and a confident conclusion of CHM's efficacy and safety for chronic cough was not possible.

Identification of Clinical Studies

The initial database search identified 15,142 potentially relevant citations. After removing duplicates and screening abstracts, 1,247 full text articles were retrieved for detailed examination. Finally, 193 RCTs, seven non-randomised controlled clinical trials (CCTs) and 12 non-controlled studies were identified (Fig. 5.1). Among them, 180 studies related to CVA, 14 studies related to UACS and 18 studies related to GORD-C. All the studies were conducted in China.

For CVA, a total of 166 were RCTs, six were CCTs and eight were non-controlled studies. A total of 16,017 participants were evaluated in these studies. Duration of CVA ranged from eight weeks to 13 years and treatment duration ranged from five days to 14 weeks. Oral CHM was administered in 180 of the CVA studies.

Upper airway cough syndrome was assessed in 14 studies, 11 RCTs, one CCT and two non-controlled studies, including 1,408 participants. Participants had UACS symptoms for between two months to ten years. Oral CHM was used in all studies and treatment duration ranged from two to four weeks. Finally, GORD-C was assessed in 16 RCTs and two non-controlled studies, with 1,333 participants. Participants had GORD-C symptoms for between two months and 13 years. Oral CHM was used in all studies and treatment duration ranged from two to 12 weeks. The small number of UACS and GORD-C studies is likely due to less well-defined diagnosis, newer classifications and variability in participants, making it difficult to conduct clinical trials on these topics.

Evidence from RCTs was pooled in meta-analyses to provide evidence for CHM treatments, with the same approach used for non-RCTs. Other study types, such as case series, are summarised but their results are not included in evidence analysis.

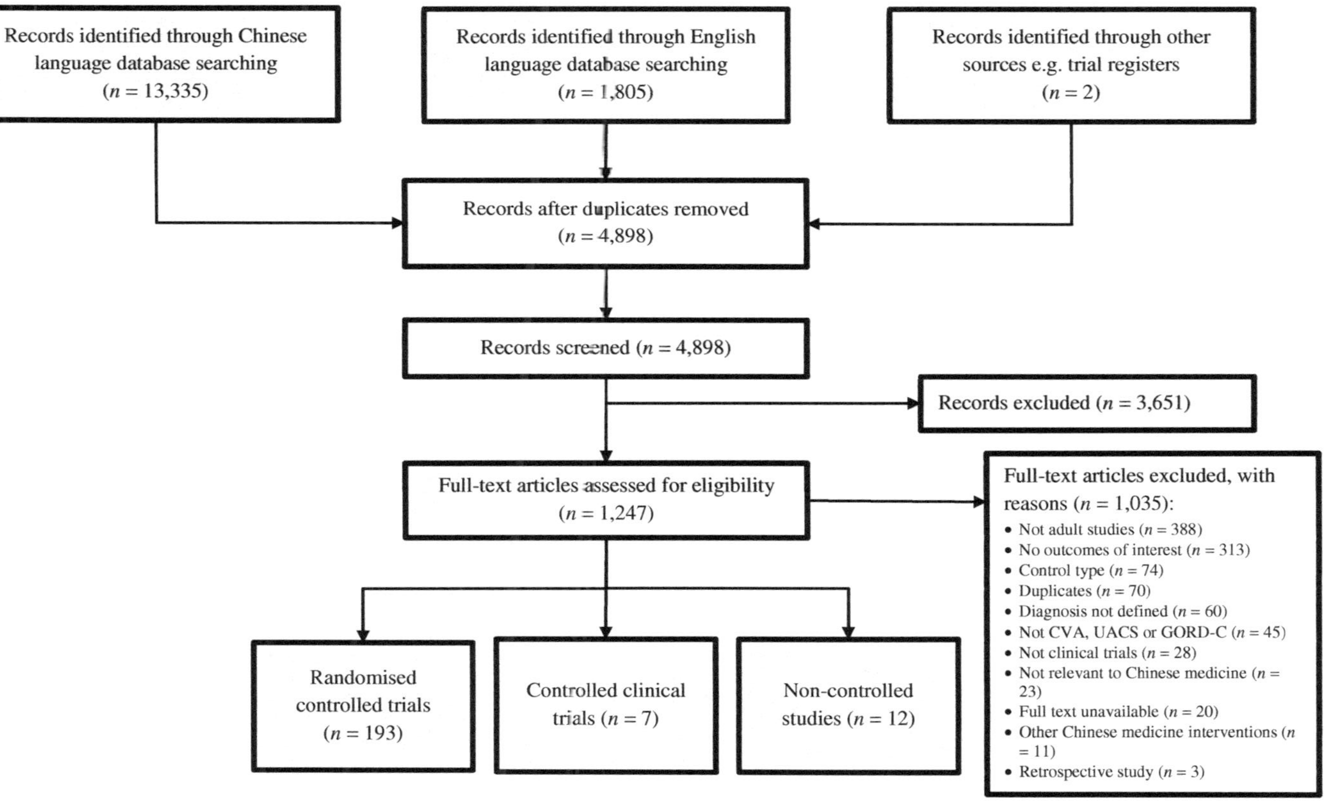

Fig. 5.1. Flowchart of study selection process: Chinese herbal medicine for chronic cough.

Chinese Herbal Medicine for Cough Variant Asthma

Chinese herbal medicine for CVA was researched in 180 studies. The results of these studies are analysed and discussed in separate sections below for the 166 RCTs (H1–H166), the six CCTs (H167–H172), and the eight non-controlled studies (H173–H180).

Randomised Controlled Trials of Chinese Herbal Medicine for Cough Variant Asthma

All 166 RCTs (H1–H166) were conducted in China. The RCTs enrolled 14,412 participants for between ten days and 14 weeks. Chinese medicine syndrome classification was used in 75 studies. The most frequently reported syndromes were:

- Severe wind attacking the Lungs 风盛挛急 (31 studies);
- Wind-phlegm obstructing the Lungs 风痰阻肺 (nine studies);
- Liver fire attacking the Lungs 肝火犯肺 (six studies);
- Hot-phlegm obstructing the Lungs 痰热郁肺 (five studies);
- Phlegm-dampness obstructing the Lungs 痰湿蕴肺 (five studies);
- Deficiency of *qi* and *yin* 气阴两虚 (four studies);
- Deficiency of Lung *yin* 肺阴亏虚 (four studies);
- Wind-cold attacking the Lungs 风寒袭肺 (four studies).

Herbal formulas were diverse and 115 different formulas were researched. All formulas were administered orally, with decoction, granule powder, pills or tablets. Thirty-four of the CHM interventions were self-made formulas. The formulas most frequently evaluated in the RCTs included *Su huang zhi ke fang* 苏黄止咳方 (24 studies), *Zhi sou san* 止嗽散 (nine studies), *Xiao qing long tang* 小青龙汤 (six studies), and *Wen dan tang* 温胆汤 (four studies). A further seven formulas were tested in two studies each, listed in Table 5.1. A total of 162 distinct herbs were used in the formulas and the most common were *gan cao* 甘草, *ma huang* 麻黄 and *chan tui* 蝉蜕 (Table 5.2).

Table 5.1. Frequently Reported Formulas in Randomised Controlled Trials of Cough Variant Asthma

Formula Name	No. of Studies	Ingredients
Su huang zhi ke fang 苏黄止咳方	24	*Zhi ma huang* 炙麻黄, *chan tui* 蝉蜕, *zi su ye* 紫苏叶, *zi su zi* 紫苏子, *qian hu* 前胡, *wu wei zi* 五味子, *niu bang zi* 牛蒡子, *pi pa ye* 枇杷叶 and *di long* 地龙
Zhi sou san 止嗽散	9	*Jie geng* 桔梗, *jing jie* 荆芥, *zi wan* 紫菀, *bai bu* 百部, *bai qian* 白前, *gan cao* 甘草 and *chen pi* 陈皮
Xiao qing long tang 小青龙汤	6	*Ma huang* 麻黄, *gui zhi* 桂枝, *shao yao* 芍药, *gan cao* 甘草, *gan jiang* 干姜, *xi xin* 细辛, *ban xia* 半夏 and *wu wei zi* 五味子
Wen dan tang 温胆汤	4	*Fa ban xia* 法半夏, *zhu ru* 竹茹, *zhi shi* 枳实, *chen pi* 陈皮, *fu ling* 茯苓 and *gan cao* 甘草
Yu ping feng san 玉屏风散	2	*Fang feng* 防风, *huang qi* 黄芪 and *bai zhu* 白术
Qu feng xuan fei fang 祛风宣肺方	2	*Zhi ma huang* 炙麻黄, *qian hu* 前胡, *hou po* 厚朴 and *zi wan* 紫菀
San ao tang 三拗汤	2	*Ma huang* 麻黄, *gan cao* 甘草 and *xing ren* 杏仁
Ming ke jian 敏咳煎	2	*Xuan shen* 玄参, *zhi ma huang* 炙麻黄, *wu wei zi* 五味子, *fang feng* 防风, *gou teng* 钩藤, *di long* 地龙 and *jiang can* 僵蚕
Guo ming jian 过敏煎	2	*Fang feng* 防风, *yin chai hu* 银柴胡, *bai zhi* 白芷, *wu mei* 乌梅, *gan cao* 甘草, *wu wei zi* 五味子, *chan tui* 蝉蜕, *jing jie* 荆芥 and *bai qian* 白前
Ning fei wan 宁肺丸	2	*Wu mei* 乌梅 and *ying su ke* 罂粟壳
Zhi ke jiao nang 止咳胶囊	2	*Dang shen* 党参, *mai dong* 麦冬, *wu wei zi* 五味子, *tai zi shen* 太子参, *sha shen* 沙参, *jie geng* 桔梗, *bai qian* 白前, *xing ren* 杏仁, *chuan bei* 川贝, *qian hu* 前胡, *bai bu* 百部, *kuan dong hua* 款冬花, *su zi* 苏子, *lu gen* 芦根, *zhi ke* 枳壳, *bai xian pi* 白鲜皮 and *gan cao* 甘草

1. Ingredients are referenced to the original studies.

2. The use of some herbs may be restricted in some countries. Readers are advised to comply with relevant regulations.

Table 5.2. Frequently Reported Herbs in Randomised Controlled Trials of Cough Variant Asthma

Most Common Herbs	Scientific Name	Frequency of Use
Gan cao 甘草, including *zhi gan cao* 炙甘草	*Glycyrrhiza* spp.	106
Ma huang 麻黄	*Ephedra sinica* Stapf	85
Chan tui 蝉蜕	*Cryptotympana pustulata* Fabricius	75
Xing ren 杏仁	*Prunus armeniaca* L. var. *ansu* Maxim.	73
Di long 地龙	*Pheretima* spp.	67
Jie geng 桔梗	*Platycodon grandiflorum* (Jacq.) A. DC.	63
Wu wei zi 五味子	*Schisandra chinensis* (Turcz.) Baill.	54
Zi wan 紫菀	*Aster tataricus* L. f.	48
Qian hu 前胡	*Peucedanum praeruptorum* Dunn	43
Zi su ye 紫苏叶	*Perilla frutescens* (L.) Britt. (leaf)	43
Bai bu 百部	*Stemona* spp.	42
Ban xia 半夏	*Pinellia ivaric* (Thunb.) Breit.	40
Chen pi 陈皮	*Citrus reticulata* Blanco	40
Huang qin 黄芩	*Scutellaria baicalensis* Georgi	37
Jing jie 荆芥	*Schizonepeta tenuifolia* Briq.	35
Fang feng 防风	*Saposhnikovia ivaricate* (Turcz.) Schischk.	34
Zi su zi 紫苏子	*Perilla frutescens* (L.) Britt. (fruit)	34
Jiang can 僵蚕	*Bombyx mori* Linnaeus	28
Niu bang zi 牛蒡子	*Arctium lappa* L.	27
Fu ling 茯苓	*Poria cocos* (Schw.) Wolf	26

The use of some herbs, such as *ma huang* 麻黄, may be restricted in some countries. Readers are advised to comply with relevant regulations.

Risk of Bias

All studies specified that 'randomisation' was used in the allocation of participants to the CHM intervention or the control groups. However, most of the studies did not clearly specify the method of random sequence generation (59.0%) and a small percentage (1.8%)

used a method that puts them at 'high' risk of bias, such as allocation based on the visiting order of the participants. Four studies described the method of allocation concealment (2.4%) and were assessed as 'low' risk of bias, and other studies were judged to be at 'unclear' risk. Only one study was evaluated as 'low' risk of bias in the blinding of participants and personnel because CHM placebo was used as the comparator. Other studies lacked information about blinding of participants and personnel and were at 'high' risk of bias. All studies did not specify the information of blinding of outcome assessors and included participant-reported outcomes, so they were assessed as 'high' risk.

Incomplete outcome data were assessed as 'low' risk bias if there was no missing data or drop-outs were balanced between groups. Only a small proportion of studies had incomplete outcome data (1.2%) and it appeared unlikely that the others could have complete outcome data, so the majority (96.4%) were considered to be at 'low' risk. Study protocols were not identified for any of the studies (either in electronic databases or clinical trial registries); therefore, most studies were assessed as 'unclear' risk of bias for selective reporting. In summary, the methodological quality was 'low' to 'moderate', and results should be interpreted with caution because none of the studies were free from bias. The risk of bias is summarised in Table 5.3.

Table 5.3.   Risk of Bias of Randomised Controlled Trials: Cough Variant Asthma

Risk of Bias Domain	Low Risk *n* (%)	Unclear Risk *n* (%)	High Risk *n* (%)
Sequence generation	65 (39.2)	98 (59.0)	3 (1.8)
Allocation concealment	4 (2.4)	162 (97.6)	0 (0.0)
Blinding of participants	1 (0.6)	0 (0.0)	165 (99.4)
Blinding of personnel	1 (0.6)	0 (0.0)	165 (99.4)
Blinding of outcome assessors	0 (0.0)	0 (0.0)	166 (100.0)
Incomplete outcome data	160 (96.4)	4 (2.4)	2 (1.2)
Selective outcome reporting	0 (0.0)	164 (98.8)	2 (1.2)

Outcomes

Outcomes included the Leicester cough questionnaire (LCQ);[10] cough symptom score;[11–13] visual analogue scale (VAS); lung function including forced expiratory volume-one second (FEV_1), forced vital capacity (FVC) and peak expiratory flow (PEF); exhaled nitric oxide (FeNO),[14] eosinophil cationic protein (ECP), blood eosinophil count (EOS), cough reflex sensitivity[15] and total effective rate.[16–17] The most common outcome was effective rate reported in 152 studies, followed by lung function FEV_1 in 50 studies, PEF in 41 studies and FVC in 20 studies. Blood eosinophil count was reported in 41 studies, cough symptom score in 29 studies, LCQ in 10 studies, VAS in nine studies, ECP in six studies, FeNO in four studies and cough reflex sensitivity in one study. Adverse events were reported in 60 studies.

In the following sections, the meta-analysis results are presented according to the outcome measure. For each outcome, studies are grouped by the comparator; for instance, CHM versus placebo, CHM versus pharmacotherapies, CHM plus pharmacotherapies versus pharmacotherapies alone as integrative medicine. Subgroup analysis included studies with low risk of bias for sequence generation, treatment duration (less than or equal to four weeks and greater than four weeks), CM syndrome classification (i.e. specified in greater than or equal to 5 studies) and CHM formula (i.e. specified in greater than or equal to five studies). The pre-specified subgroup analyses were conducted to explore heterogeneity.

Leicester Cough Questionnaire

Ten of the 166 studies used the LCQ to assess health-related quality of life in 721 participants. Meta-analysis for LCQ was performed at the end of treatment based on different comparators.

Chinese Herbal Medicine versus Pharmacotherapy

Eight RCTs ($n = 633$) compared CHM with pharmacotherapy. Two classes of drugs were used as comparators, including inhaled corticosteroids (ICS) plus bronchodilators and montelukast. Treatment

Table 5.4. Chinese Herbal Medicine versus Pharmacotherapy: Leicester Cough Questionnaire

Descriptor	No. of Studies (Participants)	Effect Size (MD [95% CI], I^2)	Included Studies
Pharmacotherapy	8 (633)	1.71 [0.55, 2.83]*, 97.4%	H18, H72, H75, H102, H120, H126, H129, H148
Sequence generation: 'low' risk of bias	7 (573)	1.58 [0.38, 2.78]*, 97.7%	H18, H72, H75, H102, H120, H129, H148
Treatment duration ≤ four weeks	7 (567)	2.04 [1.09, 2.99]*, 90.3%	H18, H72, H102, H120, H126, H129, H148
Inhaled corticosteroids plus bronchodilator	2 (127)	0.41 [–0.73, 1.56], 79.5%	H75, H102
Montelukast	5 (345)	2.23 [0.81, 3.65]*, 86.9%	H18, H72, H120, H126, H129

*Statistically significant; see Chapter 4.
Abbreviations: CI, confidence interval; MD, mean difference.

duration ranged from two to six weeks. 'Low' risk of bias for sequence generation, treatment duration and syndrome classification were used as variables in subgroup analysis. Results indicated that LCQ scores in participants receiving CHM were better than the pharmacotherapy group, but heterogeneity was high (mean difference [MD]: 1.71 points [0.55, 2.83]; I^2 = 97.4%) (Table 5.4).

Subgroup analysis

Subgroup analysis of seven studies (n = 573) that were judged at 'low' risk of bias for sequence generation was performed. The pooled result indicated that CHM was superior to pharmacotherapy, although heterogeneity remained 'high' (MD: 1.58 points [0.38, 2.78]; I^2 = 97.7%). Treatment duration for four weeks or less was reported in seven studies (n = 567); the result showed that CHM was better than pharmacotherapy, although heterogeneity remained 'high' (MD: 2.04 points [1.09, 2.99], I^2 = 90.3%). Subgroup analysis by drug class of

ICS plus bronchodilator showed no difference between CHM combined with ICS plus bronchodilator, compared to ICS plus bronchodilator alone in two studies (MD: 0.41 points [–0.73, 1.56], I^2 = 79.5%). Montelukast was used as the comparator in five RCTs, including 345 participants. The results indicated that CHM was superior to montelukast, although the heterogeneity was 'high' (MD: 2.23 points [0.81, 3.65]; I^2 = 86.9%).

Chinese Herbal Medicine plus Pharmacotherapy versus Pharmacotherapy

Two RCTs (H3, H149) (*n* = 88) compared CHM plus pharmacotherapy with pharmacotherapy alone. Treatment duration ranged from ten days to two weeks. Participants receiving CHM plus pharmacotherapy reported improved LCQ scores compared to pharmacotherapy alone (MD: 2.69 points [2.19, 3.18]; I^2 = 0.0%).

Cough Symptom Score

Twenty-four of the 166 studies, including 1,767 participants, assessed cough symptom score. Overall meta-analysis for cough symptom score was performed at the end of treatment based on different comparators.

Chinese Herbal Medicine versus Placebo

One RCT (H101) with 72 participants compared CHM with placebo. The results showed CHM (*Qu feng xuan fei fang* 祛风宣肺方; *ma huang* 麻黄, *qian hu* 前胡, *hou po* 厚朴, *zi wan* 紫菀) was superior to placebo (MD: –1.15 points [–1.66, –0.63]).

Chinese Herbal Medicine versus Pharmacotherapy

Thirteen RCTs (*n* = 942) compared CHM with pharmacotherapy. Subgroup analysis included 'low' risk of bias for sequence generation, treatment duration, syndrome classification and formula. Four classes of pharmacotherapies were used as comparators including ICS, ICS plus bronchodilator, ICS plus other pharmacotherapy, and montelukast. Treatment duration ranged from two to 12 weeks.

Table 5.5. Chinese Herbal Medicine versus Pharmacotherapy: Cough Symptom Score

Descriptor	No. of Studies (Participants)	Effect Size (MD/SMD [95% CI], I^2)	Included Studies
Pharmacotherapy	13 (942)	SMD –0.60 [–0.91, –0.29]*, 80.6%	H19, H72, H89, H95, H104, H120, H123, H124, H132, H133, H162, H163, H166
'Low' risk of bias: Sequence generation	7 (529)	SMD –0.86 [–1.19, –0.54]*, 67.6%	H72, H95, H120, H124, H132, H133, H163
Treatment duration: ≤ four weeks	8 (553)	SMD –0.50 [–0.97, –0.02]*, 86.2%	H72, H89, H95, H120, H123, H132, H162, H166
Treatment duration: > four weeks	5 (389)	SMD –0.73 [–1.07, –0.40]*, 59.1%	H19, H104, H124, H133, H163
Syndrome: Severe wind attacking the Lungs	3 (176)	MD –0.47 [–0.82, –0.12]*, 56.1%	H19, H95, H163
Formula: *Su huang zhi ke fang* 苏黄止咳方	3 (218)	MD –0.04 [–0.65, 0.55], 88.5%	H89, H123, H162, H166
ICS plus bronchodilator	5 (369)	SMD –0.25 [–0.89, 0.39], 88.8%	H19, H124, H133, H162, H166
Montelukast	6 (454)	MD –0.61 [–0.76, –0.45]*, 19.6%	H72, H89, H95, H104, H120, H132

*Statistically significant; see Chapter 4.
Abbreviations: CI, confidence interval; ICS, inhaled corticosteroids; MD, mean difference; SMD, standardised mean difference.

The overall result indicated that participants receiving CHM had less cough symptoms than those receiving pharmacotherapy, but heterogeneity was high (standardised mean difference [SMD] –0.60 points [–0.91, –0.29]; I^2 = 80.6%) (Table 5.5).

Subgroup analysis

Subgroup analysis by 'low' risk of bias for sequence generation
Subgroup analysis of seven studies (n = 529) that were judged at 'low'

risk of bias for sequence generation was performed. The pooled result indicated that CHM was superior to pharmacotherapy, although heterogeneity remained high (SMD: –0.86 points [–1.19, –0.54]; I^2 = 67.6%).

Subgroup analysis by treatment duration Treatment duration for four weeks or less was reported in eight studies (n = 553). The results showed that CHM was better than pharmacotherapy, although heterogeneity remained 'high' (SMD: –0.50 points [–0.97, –0.02], I^2 = 86.2%). Five RCTs including 389 participants, with treatment duration longer than four weeks, also showed that CHM was superior to pharmacotherapy, although heterogeneity was substantial (SMD: –0.73 points [–1.07, –0.40]; I^2 = 59.1%).

Subgroup analysis by syndrome classification Syndrome classification of severe wind attacking the Lungs was reported in three RCTs (n = 176). The result indicated that cough symptom score decreased in participants receiving CHM, compared to pharmacotherapy, although heterogeneity was 'high' (MD: –0.47 points [–0.82, –0.12]; I^2 = 56.1%).

Subgroup analysis by formula The formula *Su huang zhi ke fang* 苏黄止咳方 was used in three RCTs (n = 218) and it was not superior to pharmacotherapy (MD: –0.04 points [–0.65, 0.55]; I^2 = 88.5%).

Subgroup analysis by comparator drug class Inhaled corticosteroids plus bronchodilator was used as comparator in five RCTs (n = 369). The pooled result indicated that there was no difference between CHM and ICS plus bronchodilator (SMD: –0.25 points [–0.89, 0.39]; I^2 = 88.8%). Montelukast was used as comparator in six RCTs, including 454 participants. The results indicated that CHM was superior to montelukast, and the heterogeneity was 'low' (MD: –0.61 points [–0.76, –0.45]; I^2 = 19.6%).

Chinese Herbal Medicine plus Pharmacotherapy versus Pharmacotherapy Alone

Twelve RCTs (n = 811) compared CHM plus pharmacotherapy with pharmacotherapy alone. Treatment duration ranged from one to 12 weeks. The overall result indicated that cough symptoms were reduced in participants receiving CHM plus pharmacotherapy, compared to pharmacotherapy alone, but heterogeneity was 'high' (SMD: −1.79 points [−2.47, −1.12]; I^2 = 94.0%) (Table 5.6).

Table 5.6. Chinese Herbal Medicine plus Pharmacotherapy versus Pharmacotherapy: Cough Symptom Score

Descriptor	No. of Studies (Participants)	Effect Size (MD/SMD [95% CI], I^2)	Included Studies
Pharmacotherapy	12 (811)	SMD −1.79 [−2.47, −1.12]*, 94.0%	H2, H16, H28, H29, H44, H56, H57, H91, H121, H149, H162, H166
'Low' risk of bias: Sequence generation	5 (334)	SMD −1.59 [−2.58, −0.60]*, 93.4%	H28, H56, H57, H121, H149
Treatment duration: ≤ four weeks	9 (592)	SMD −2.10 [−3.02, −1.18]*, 95.1%	H2, H28, H29, H44, H57, H121, H149, H162, H166
Treatment duration: > four weeks	3 (219)	SMD −1.79 [−2.47, −1.12]*, 70.2%	H16, H56, H91
Syndrome differentiation: Wind-phlegm obstructing the Lungs	2 (117)	SMD −0.73 [−1.11, −0.36]*, 0.0%	H28, H91
Formula: Su huang zhi ke fang 苏黄止咳方	3 (202)	MD −1.08 [−1.78, −0.37]*, 95.6%	H29, H162, H166
ICS plus bronchodilator	6 (394)	SMD −1.24 [−1.76, −0.73]*, 81.3%	H16, H28, H56, H149, H162, H166
ICS plus other pharmacotherapy	7 (451)	SMD −1.16 [−1.61, −0.70]*, 79.7%	H16, H28, H56, H91, H149, H162, H166

*Statistically significant; see Chapter 4.

Abbreviations: CI, confidence interval; ICS, inhaled corticosteroids; MD, mean difference; SMD, standardised mean difference.

Subgroup analysis

Subgroup analysis by 'low' risk of bias for sequence generation
Subgroup analysis of five studies (n = 334) that were judged at 'low' risk of bias for sequence generation was performed. The pooled result indicated that CHM plus pharmacotherapy was superior to pharmacotherapy, and heterogeneity remained 'high' (SMD: −1.59 points [−2.58, −0.60]; I^2 = 93.4%).

Subgroup analysis by treatment duration Treatment duration for four weeks or less was reported in nine studies (n = 592). The results showed that CHM plus pharmacotherapy was better than pharmacotherapy alone, although heterogeneity remained 'high' (SMD: −2.10 points [−3.02, −1.18], I^2 = 95.1%). Three RCTs including 219 participants, with treatment duration longer than four weeks; also showed CHM plus pharmacotherapy was superior to pharmacotherapy alone, although heterogeneity was 'high' (SMD: −1.79 points [−2.47, −1.12]; I^2 = 70.2%).

Subgroup analysis by syndrome classification Syndrome classification wind-phlegm obstructing the Lungs was assessed in two studies (n = 117). The result of analysis showed participants with wind-phlegm obstructing the Lungs receiving CHM plus pharmacotherapy was superior to pharmacotherapy alone, and heterogeneity was 'low' (SMD: −0.73 points [−1.11, −0.36]; I^2 = 0.0%).

Subgroup analysis by formula *Su huang zhi ke fang* 苏黄止咳方 was assessed in three studies (n = 202) and, combined with pharmacotherapy, it was superior to pharmacotherapy alone (MD: −1.08 points [−1.78, −0.37]; I^2 = 95.6%).

Subgroup analysis by drug class Inhaled corticosteroids plus bronchodilator was used as comparator in six RCTs (n = 394). The pooled result indicated that CHM plus ICS and bronchodilator was superior to ICS plus bronchodilator alone (SMD: −1.24 points [−1.76, −0.73]; I^2 = 81.3%). Furthermore, ICS plus other pharmacotherapy was used as comparator in seven RCTs (n = 451). The results indicated CHM combined with ICS plus other pharmacotherapy was superior to ICS plus other pharmacotherapy alone (SMD: –1.16 points [–1.61, –0.70]; I^2 = 79.7%).

Visual Analogue Scale

Nine of the 166 studies (*n* = 620) assessed VAS. Overall meta-analysis for VAS was performed at the end of treatment based on different comparators.

Chinese Herbal Medicine versus Placebo

One RCT (H101) with 72 participants compared CHM to placebo. The results showed CHM (*Qu feng xuan fei fang* 祛风宣肺方) was superior to placebo (MD: –1.76 points [–2.65, –0.86]).

Chinese Herbal Medicine versus Pharmacotherapy

Six RCTs (*n* = 407) compared CHM with pharmacotherapy. Treatment duration ranged from two to six weeks. The meta-analysis result indicated that participants receiving CHM had reduced cough symptoms compared to participants taking pharmacotherapy, but heterogeneity was 'high' (MD: –0.68 points [–1.32, –0.04]; I^2 = 69.1%) (Table 5.7).

Subgroup analysis

Subgroup analysis by 'low' risk of bias for sequence generation Subgroup analysis of two studies (*n* = 129) that were judged at 'low' risk of bias for sequence generation was performed. The pooled result indicated that there was no difference between CHM and pharmacotherapy (MD: –0.27 points [–1.18, 0.62]; I^2 = 58.1%).

Subgroup analysis by treatment duration Treatment duration for four weeks or less was reported in five studies (*n* = 341). The results showed that CHM was not better than pharmacotherapy (MD: –0.68 points [–1.50, 0.13]; I^2 = 75.3%).

Table 5.7. Chinese Herbal Medicine versus Pharmacotherapy: Visual Analogue Scale

Descriptor	No. of Studies (Participants)	Effect Size (MD [95% CI], I^2)	Included Studies
Pharmacotherapy	6 (407)	–0.68 [–1.32, –0.04]*, 69.1%	H45, H75, H81, H112, H139, H166
'Low' risk of bias: Sequence generation	2 (129)	–0.27 [–1.18, 0.62], 58.1%	H75, H81
Treatment duration: ≤ four weeks	5 (341)	–0.68 [–1.50, 0.13], 75.3%	H45, H81, H112, H139, H166
Syndrome classification: Wind-phlegm obstructing the Lungs	2 (127)	–0.51 [–2.01, 0.98], 78.7%	H81, H139
ICS plus bronchodilator	5 (347)	–0.66 [–1.48, 0.15], 74.9%	H45, H75, H81, H139, H166

*Statistically significant; see Chapter 4.

Abbreviations: CI, confidence interval; ICS, inhaled corticosteroids; MD, mean difference.

Subgroup analysis by syndrome classification Scores for VAS were not statistically significant between groups when studies were subgrouped by syndrome classification, wind-phlegm obstructing the Lungs (MD: –0.51 points [–2.01, 0.98]; I^2 = 78.7%).

Subgroup analysis by drug class Inhaled corticosteroids plus bronchodilator was used as comparator in five RCTs (n = 347). The pooled result indicated that there was no difference between groups (MD: –0.66 points [–1.48, 0.15]; I^2 = 74.9%).

Chinese Herbal Medicine plus Pharmacotherapy versus Pharmacotherapy Alone

Three RCTs (n = 170) compared CHM plus pharmacotherapy with pharmacotherapy alone. Treatment duration ranged from ten days to four weeks. Meta-analysis showed that cough symptoms improved in

Table 5.8. Chinese Herbal Medicine plus Pharmacotherapy versus Pharmacotherapy Alone: Visual Analogue Scale

Descriptor	No. of Studies (Participants)	Effect Size (MD [95% CI], I^2)	Included Studies
Pharmacotherapy	3 (170)	–1.20 [–1.66, –0.75]*, 24.7%	H21, H149, H166
Low risk of bias: Sequence generation	2 (108)	–1.09 [–1.80, –0.38]*, 56.4%	H21, H149
ICS plus bronchodilator	2 (110)	–1.42 [–1.87, –0.96]*, 0.0%	H149, H166

*Statistically significant; see Chapter 4.
Abbreviations: CI, confidence interval; ICS, inhaled corticosteroids; MD, mean difference.

participants receiving CHM plus pharmacotherapy, compared to pharmacotherapy alone, and heterogeneity was 'low' (MD: –1.20 points [–1.66, –0.75]; I^2 = 24.7%) (Table 5.8).

Subgroup analysis

Two studies (n = 108) were judged at 'low' risk of bias for sequence generation. The pooled result indicated that CHM plus pharmacotherapy was superior to pharmacotherapy alone, although heterogeneity was 'high' (MD: –1.09 points [–1.80, –0.38]; I^2 = 56.4%). Subgroup analysis of two studies by drug class of ICS plus bronchodilator (n = 110), indicated that CHM plus pharmacotherapy was superior to ICS plus bronchodilator alone, and heterogeneity was 'low' (MD: –1.42 points [–1.87, –0.96]; I^2 = 0.0%).

Lung Function: Forced Expiratory Volume in One Second

Forty-nine of the 166 studies (including 4,517 participants) assessed FEV_1. Thirty-two studies reported FEV_1 litres (L) and 17 reported FEV_1 percentage (%). Overall meta-analysis for FEV_1 was performed at the end of treatment based on different comparators.

Chinese Herbal Medicine versus Pharmacotherapy

Nineteen RCTs (n = 1,561) compared CHM with pharmacotherapy. Treatment duration ranged from one to four weeks. The FEV_1 L was increased in participants receiving CHM compared to pharmacotherapy, although heterogeneity was 'high' (MD: 0.26 L [0.05, 0.48]; I^2 = 93.5%); FEV_1% was also improved (MD: 5.73% [2.37, 9.08]; I^2 = 93.4%) (Table 5.9).

Table 5.9. Chinese Herbal Medicine versus Pharmacotherapy: Forced Expiratory Volume in One Second

Descriptor	No. of Studies (Participants)	Effect Size (MD [95% CI], I^2)	Included Studies
Pharmacotherapy for FEV_1 L	9 (819)	0.26 [0.05, 0.48]*, 93.5%	H51, H86, H90, H98, H110, H111, H127, H138, H144
Pharmacotherapy for FEV_1%	10 (742)	5.73 [2.37, 9.08]*, 93.4%	H35, H38, H63, H70, H88, H94, H132, H157, H160, H161
'Low' risk of bias: Sequence generation FEV_1L	3 (249)	0.08 [−0.14, 0.30], 73%	H86, H110, H144
'Low' risk of bias: Sequence generation FEV_1%	5 (382)	2.70 [0.72, 4.67]*, 0.0%	H63, H94, H132, H160, H161
Treatment duration: ≤ four weeks FEV_1%	9 (682)	6.40 [2.98, 9.83], 93.6%	H35, H38, H63, H70, H88, H94, H132, H157, H160
ICS plus bronchodilator FEV_1L	2 (238)	−0.01 [−0.11, 0.09], 0.0%	H111, H144
ICS plus bronchodilator FEV_1%	3 (204)	3.12 [1.38, 4.85]*, 0.0%	H88, H160, H161
ICS plus other pharmacotherapy FEV_1L	3 (299)	−0.01 [−0.10, 0.07], 0.0%	H110, H111, H144
ICS plus other pharmacotherapy FEV_1%	4 (304)	3.13 [1.47, 4.79]*, 0.0%	H88, H94, H160, H161

*Statistically significant; see Chapter 4.

Abbreviations: CI, confidence interval; FEV_1, forced expiratory volume in one second; ICS, inhaled corticosteroids; L, litres; MD, mean difference.

Subgroup analysis

Subgroup analysis by 'low' risk of bias for sequence generation For FEV_1 L, subgroup analysis of three studies ($n = 249$) that were judged at 'low' risk of bias for sequence generation was performed. There were no differences between CHM and pharmacotherapy (MD: 0.08 L [–0.14, 0.30]; $I^2 = 73\%$). For $FEV_1\%$, subgroup analysis of five studies ($n = 382$) that were judged at 'low' risk of bias for sequence generation was performed. The pooled result showed CHM was superior to pharmacotherapy, and heterogeneity decreased significantly (MD: 2.7% [0.72, 4.67]; $I^2 = 0.0\%$).

Subgroup analysis by treatment duration All studies evaluating FEV_1 L had a treatment duration less than, or equal to, four weeks, and subgrouping was not appropriate. Nine out of the ten studies evaluating $FEV_1\%$ had a treatment duration of four weeks or less ($n = 682$); pooled results favoured CHM compared to pharmacotherapy (MD: 6.40% [2.98, 9.83]; $I^2 = 93.6\%$).

Subgroup analysis by syndrome classification The three studies that used syndrome classification included participants with different syndromes; therefore the results could not be merged in meta-analysis.

Subgroup analysis by formula Studies evaluated different formula and therefore results could not be pooled in meta-analysis.

Subgroup analysis by drug class Inhaled corticosteroids plus bronchodilator was used as the comparator in two RCTs ($n = 238$) evaluating FEV_1 L and three RCTs ($n = 204$) evaluating $FEV_1\%$. FEV_1 L was not statistically significant between groups (MD: –0.01 L [–0.11, 0.09]; $I^2 = 0.0\%$), but CHM was superior to ICS plus bronchodilator in terms of $FEV_1\%$, and heterogeneity was 'low' (MD: 3.12% [1.38, 4.85]; $I^2 = 0.0\%$). Inhaled corticosteroids plus other pharmacotherapy was used as comparator in three RCTs ($n = 299$) with FEV_1 L and four RCTs ($n = 304$) with $FEV_1\%$. The result indicated that CHM was not superior to ICS plus other pharmacotherapies (MD: –0.01 L [–0.10, 0.07]; $I^2 = 0.0\%$), but CHM was superior to ICS plus other pharmacotherapies in terms of $FEV_1\%$, and heterogeneity was 'low' (MD: 3.13% [1.47, 4.79]; $I^2 = 0.0\%$). Montelukast was only evaluated in one study and pooling in meta-analysis was not appropriate.

Chinese Herbal Medicine plus Pharmacotherapy versus Pharmacotherapy Alone

Thirty-one RCTs (*n* = 3,096) compared CHM plus pharmacotherapy with pharmacotherapy alone. Treatment duration ranged from ten days to eight weeks. The overall result indicated that FEV_1L increased in participants receiving CHM plus pharmacotherapy, compared to pharmacotherapy alone, although heterogeneity was 'high' (MD: 0.36 L [0.20, 0.52]; I^2 = 96.1%). The effect was also seen in FEV_1% (MD: 8.04% [6.49, 10.32]; I^2 = 71.5%) (Table 5.10). The results of subgroup analyses are shown in Table 5.11.

Subgroup analysis

Subgroup analysis by 'low' risk of bias for sequence generation For FEV_1 L, subgroup analysis of seven studies (*n* = 586) that were judged

Table 5.10. Chinese Herbal Medicine plus Pharmacotherapy versus Pharmacotherapy Alone: Forced Expiratory Volume in One Second

Descriptor	No. of Studies (Participants)	Effect Size (MD [95% CI], I^2)	Included Studies
Pharmacotherapy for FEV_1 L	23 (2,214)	0.36 [0.20, 0.52]*, 96.1%	H3, H5, H6, H17, H23, H29, H37, H54, H64, H84, H91, H96, H97, H100, H119, H136, H143, H150, H151, H154, H156, H159, H164
Pharmacotherapy for FEV_1%	9 (882)	8.04 [6.49, 10.32]*, 71.5%	H28, H33, H34, H59, H77, H92, H151, H160, H161

*Statistically significant; see Chapter 4.

Abbreviations: CI, confidence interval; FEV_1, forced expiratory volume in one second; L, litres; MD, mean difference.

Table 5.11. Subgroup Analysis for Forced Expiratory Volume in One Second

Subgroup	Category	No. of Studies (Participants)	Effect Size (MD [95% CI], I^2)	Included Studies
'Low' risk of bias: Sequence generation FEV_1 L	Low RoB	7 (586)	0.36 [0.22, 0.50]*, 87.1%	H3, H5, H17, H37, H100, H143, H154
'Low' risk of bias: Sequence generation FEV1%	Low RoB	3 (200)	6.70 [3.64, 9.77]*, 0.0%	H28, H160, H161
Treatment duration for FEV_1L	$\leq$ four weeks	14 (1,042)	0.41 [0.11, 0.70]*, 97.0%	H3, H5, H6, H23, H29, H54, H64, H84, H96, H100, H136, H151, H154, H159
	> four weeks	9 (900)	0.36 [0.20, 0.52]*, 82.5%	H17, H37, H91, H97, H119, H143, H150, H156, H164
Treatment duration for FEV_1%	$\leq$ four weeks	6 (662)	7.75 [4.35, 11.14]*, 78.6%	H28, H33, H34, H59, H151, H160
	> four weeks	3 (220)	9.15 [7.85, 10.45]*, 0.0%	H77, H92, H161
Syndrome classification for FEV_1L	Severe wind invading the Lungs	2 (180)	0.28 [0.03, 0.52]*, 58.1%	H23, H100
	Wind-phlegm obstructing the Lungs	2 (94)	0.08 [−0.09, 0.25], 0.0%	H6, H91
	Liver fire attacking the Lungs	2 (132)	0.34 [−0.07, 0.77], 79.6%	H3, H17
Syndrome classification for FEV_1%	Severe wind invading the Lungs	2 (116)	6.12 [2.14, 10.11]*, 0.0%	H34, H160

(Continued)

Table 5.11. (*Continued*)

Subgroup	Category	No. of Studies (Participants)	Effect Size (MD [95% CI], I^2)	Included Studies
Formula for FEV$_1$ L	Su huang zhi ke fang 苏黄止咳方	9 (953)	0.51 [0.20, 0.82]*, 98.3%	H29, H84, H96, H97, H100, H143, H154, H156, H159
	Zhi sou san 止嗽散	3 (418)	0.36 [0.25, 0.47]*, 0.0%	H119, H136, H150
Comparator drug class	ICS	2 (165)	0.79 [−0.86, 2.44], 99.2%	H29, H164
	ICS plus Bronchodilator for FEV$_1$L	9 (931)	0.30 [0.19, 0.40]*, 67.0%	H6, H17, H37, H64, H84, H100, H136, H150, H156
	ICS plus Bronchodilator for FEV$_1$%	4 (300)	8.79 [7.44, 10.14]*, 0.0%	H28, H77, H160, H161
	ICS plus other pharmacotherapy for FEV$_1$L	15 (1,357)	0.31 [0.21, 0.40]*, 76.6%	H3, H6, H17, H23, H37, H64, H84, H91, H96, H100, H119, H136, H150, H151, H156
	ICS plus other pharmacotherapy for FEV$_1$%	6 (710)	9.28 [7.38, 11.19]*, 68.7%	H28, H77, H92, H151, H160, H161
	Montelukast FEV$_1$ L)	3 (377)	0.41 [0.12, 0.69]*, 84.2%	H5, H54, H97

*Statistically significant; see Chapter 4.

Abbreviations: CI, confidence interval; FEV$_1$, forced expiratory volume in one second; ICS, inhaled corticosteroids; L, litres; MD, mean difference; RoB, risk of bias.

at 'low' risk of bias for sequence generation was performed. The pooled result showed CHM plus pharmacotherapy was superior to pharmacotherapy alone, although heterogeneity did not decrease significantly (MD: 0.36 L [0.22, 0.50]; I^2 = 87.1%) (Table 5.11). For FEV$_1$%, subgroup analysis of three studies (n = 200) that were judged at 'low' risk of bias for sequence generation was performed. The pooled result showed CHM plus pharmacotherapy was superior to pharmacotherapy alone, and heterogeneity decreased significantly (MD: 6.70% [3.64, 9.77]; $I^2 = 0.0\%$).

Subgroup analysis by treatment duration Treatment duration for four weeks or less in 14 studies ($n = 1,042$) with FEV_1 L favoured CHM plus pharmacotherapy, compared to pharmacotherapy alone, and heterogeneity remained 'high' (MD: 0.41 L [0.11, 0.70]; $I^2 = 97.0\%$). Nine RCTs, including 900 participants, with treatment duration longer than four weeks, also showed CHM plus pharmacotherapy was superior to pharmacotherapy alone (MD: 0.36 L [0.20, 0.52]; $I^2 = 82.5\%$) although heterogeneity did not decrease significantly. Treatment duration for four weeks or less in six studies ($n = 662$) with $FEV_1\%$ favoured CHM plus pharmacotherapy, compared to pharmacotherapy alone (MD: 7.75% [4.35, 11.14]; $I^2 = 78.6\%$). Three studies, including 220 participants, with treatment duration longer than four weeks, showed CHM plus pharmacotherapy was better than pharmacotherapy alone in terms of $FEV_1\%$, and heterogeneity was 'low' (MD: 9.15% [7.85, 10.45]; $I^2 = 0.0\%$).

Subgroup analysis by syndrome classification Syndrome classification was used in six RCTs. The pooled result of the subgroups showed that 180 participants in two studies with severe wind attacking the Lungs receiving CHM plus pharmacotherapy was superior to pharmacotherapy alone, although heterogeneity was substantial (MD: 0.28 L [0.03, 0.52]; $I^2 = 58.1\%$). There was no difference between CHM plus pharmacotherapy and pharmacotherapy alone in participants with wind-phlegm obstructing the Lungs (MD: 0.08 L [–0.09, 0.25]; $I^2 = 0.0\%$) or Liver fire attacking the Lungs (MD: 0.34 L [–0.07, 0.77]; $I^2 = 79.6\%$).

In terms of $FEV_1\%$, syndrome classification was used in four RCTs. The pooled result of subgroup showed participants with severe wind attacking the Lungs receiving CHM plus pharmacotherapy was superior to pharmacotherapy, and heterogeneity was 'low' (MD: 6.12% [2.14, 10.11]; $I^2 = 0.0\%$).

Subgroup analysis by formula *Su huang zhi ke fang* 苏黄止咳方 plus pharmacotherpy was used in nine studies ($n = 953$); it was superior to pharmacotherapy alone, although heterogeneity remained 'high' in the subgroup (MD: 0.51 L [0.20, 0.82]; I^2 = 98.3%). *Zhi sou san* 止嗽散 was evaluated in three studies (*n* = 418). *Zhi sou san* 止嗽散 plus pharmacotherpy was superior to pharmacotherapy alone, and the heterogeneity was 'low' (MD: 0.36 L [0.25, 0.47]; I^2 = 0.0%).

Subgroup analysis by drug class Inhaled corticosteroids was used as comparator in two RCTs (*n* = 165) and the pooled result indicated that there was no difference between CHM plus ICS compared to ICS alone (MD: 0.79 L [–0.86, 2.44]; I^2 = 99.2%). Inhaled corticosteroids plus bronchodilator was used as comparator in nine RCTs (*n* = 931) evaluating FEV_1 L and four RCTs (*n* = 300) evaluating FEV_1%. The pooled result of FEV_1 L indicated that CHM combined with ICS and bronchodilator was superior to ICS plus bronchodilator alone (MD: 0.30 L [0.19, 0.40]; I^2 = 67.0%). The effect was also seen for FEV_1% (MD: 8.79% [7.44, 10.14]; I^2 = 0.0%).

Inhaled corticosteroids plus other pharmacotherapy was used as comparator in 15 RCTs (*n* = 1,357) evaluating FEV_1 L and six RCTs (*n* = 710) evaluating FEV_1%. The pooled result of FEV_1 L indicated that CHM combined with ICS and other pharmacotherapies was superior to ICS plus other pharmacotherapies alone (MD: 0.30 litre [0.20, 0.40]; I^2 = 76.6%). The effect was also seen in terms of FEV_1% (MD: 9.28% [7.38, 11.19]; I^2 = 68.7%).

Montelukast was used as comparator in three RCTs, including 377 participants. The result indicated that CHM plus montelukast was superior to montelukast alone; however, the heterogeneity was 'high' (MD: 0.41 L [0.12, 0.69]; I^2 = 84.2%).

Lung Function: Forced Vital Capacity

Eighteen of the 166 studies (including 1,909 participants) assessed FVC. Overall meta-analysis for FVC was performed at the end of treatment based on different comparators.

Chinese Herbal Medicine versus Pharmacotherapy

Five RCTs (*n* = 348) compared CHM with pharmacotherapy. Treatment duration ranged from ten days to four weeks. The overall result indicated

Table 5.12. Chinese Herbal Medicine versus Pharmacotherapy: Forced Vital Capacity

Descriptor	No. of Studies (Participants)	Effect Size (MD [95% CI], I^2)	Included Studies
Pharmacotherapy	5 (348)	0.09 [–0.15, 0.34], 69.0%	H48, H86, H90, H160, H161
'Low' risk of bias: Sequence generation	4 (268)	–0.06 [–0.44, 0.31], 71.7%	H48, H86, H160, H161
Treatment duration: ≤ four weeks	4 (288)	0.14 [–0.11, 0.40], 70.5%	H48, H86, H90, H160
ICS plus bronchodilator	2 (140)	–0.25 [–0.59, 0.09], 0.0%	H160, H161

Abbreviations: CI, confidence interval; ICS, inhaled corticosteroids; MD, mean difference.

that the FVC of participants receiving CHM was not superior to pharmacotherapy (MD: 0.09 L [–0.15, 0.34]; I^2 = 69.0%) (Table 5.12).

Subgroup analysis

Subgroup analysis of four studies (*n* = 268) that were judged at 'low' risk of bias for sequence generation was performed. There was no difference between CHM and pharmacotherapy (MD: –0.06 L [–0.44, 0.31]; I^2 = 71.7%). Treatment duration for four weeks or less was reported in four studies (*n* = 288); there was no difference between CHM and pharmacotherapy (MD: 0.14 L [–0.11, 0.40]; I^2 = 70.5%). The CM syndromes were different in each study and therefore it could not be analysed as a subgroup. Inhaled corticosteroids plus bronchodilators was used as comparator in two RCTs (*n* = 140). The pooled result indicated that there was no difference between CHM and ICS plus bronchodilators (MD: –0.25 L [–0.59, 0.09]; I^2 = 0.0%).

Chinese Herbal Medicine plus Pharmacotherapy versus Pharmacotherapy Alone

Forced vital capacity (in litres) was measured in 14 RCTs (*n* = 1,351) that compared CHM plus pharmacotherapy with pharmacotherapy alone. Forced vital capacity % was reported in one study. Treatment duration ranged from two to eight weeks. Forced vital capacity L increased in participants receiving CHM plus pharmacotherapy, compared to pharmacotherapy alone, although heterogeneity was 'high' (MD: 0.47 L [0.28, 0.66]; I^2 = 92.8%). Forced vital capacity % also improved in the CHM integrative medicine group (MD: 6.7% [5.35, 8.04]) (Table 5.13).

Table 5.13. Chinese Herbal Medicine plus Pharmacotherapy versus Pharmacotherapy Alone: Forced Vital Capacity

Descriptor	No. of Studies (Participants)	Effect Size (MD [95% CI], I^2)	Included Studies
Pharmacotherapy	14 (1,351)	0.47 L [0.28, 0.66]*, 92.8%	H5, H17, H28, H29, H37, H43, H64, H96, H97, H100, H154, H160, H161, H164
Pharmacotherapy	1 (350)	6.7 L [5.35, 8.04]*	H59
'Low' risk of bias: Sequence generation	9 (726)	0.33% [0.16, 0.50]*, 75.6%	H5, H17, H28, H37, H43, H100, H154, H160, H161
Treatment duration: ≤ 4 weeks	9 (739)	0.53 L [0.14, 0.93]*, 94.4%	H5, H28, H29, H43, H64, H96, H100, H154, H160
Treatment duration: > 4 weeks	5 (612)	0.38 L [0.19, 0.58]*, 88.7%	H17, H37, H97, H161, H164
Syndrome classification: Severe wind invading the Lungs	3 (230)	0.13 L [–0.09, 0.37], 18.8%	H43, H100, H160
Comparator: ICS	2 (165)	1.03 L [–0.44, 2.51], 98.0%	H29, H164
Comparator: ICS plus bronchodilators	7 (622)	0.25 L [0.05, 0.45]*, 80.6%	H17, H28, H37, H64, H100, H160, H161
Comparator: ICS plus other pharmacotherapies	9 (769)	0.31 L [0.14, 0.48]*, 77.2%	H17, H28, H37, H43, H64, H96, H100, H160, H161
Comparator: Montelukast	2 (317)	0.63 L [0.57, 0.68]*, 0.0%	H5, H97

*Statistically significant; see Chapter 4.
Abbreviations: CI, confidence interval; ICS, inhaled corticosteroids; L, litres; MD, mean difference.

Subgroup analysis

Subgroup analysis of nine studies (n = 726) that were judged at 'low' risk of bias for sequence generation was performed. The pooled result showed that CHM plus pharmacotherapy was superior to pharmacotherapy alone, although heterogeneity did not decrease significantly (MD: 0.33 L [0.16, 0.50]; I^2 = 75.6%).

Treatment duration for four weeks or less in nine studies (n = 739) favoured CHM plus pharmacotherapy, compared with pharmacotherapy alone, and heterogeneity remained 'high' (MD: 0.53 L [0.14, 0.93]; I^2 = 94.4%). Five RCTs including 612 participants, with treatment duration longer than four weeks, also showed CHM plus pharmacotherapy was superior to pharmacotherapy alone (MD: 0.38 L [0.19, 0.58]; I^2 = 88.7%) although heterogeneity did not decrease significantly. The CM syndrome of severe wind invading the Lungs was assessed in three studies and the pooled results showed no difference between groups (MD 0.13 L [–0.09, 0.37]; I^2 = 18.8%).

Inhaled corticosteroids was used as comparator in two RCTs, including 165 participants. The result indicated that there was no difference between CHM plus ICS and ICS alone (MD: 1.03 L [–0.44, 2.51]; I^2 = 98.0%). Inhaled corticosteroids plus bronchodilators was used as the comparator in seven RCTs (n = 622). The pooled result indicated that CHM combined with ICS and bronchodilators was superior to ICS plus bronchodilators alone (MD: 0.25 L [0.05, 0.45]; I^2 = 80.6%). Inhaled corticosteroids plus other pharmacotherapies was used as the comparator in nine RCTs (n = 769). The pooled result of FVC (L) indicated that CHM as integrative medicine was superior to ICS plus other pharmacotherapies alone (MD: 0.31 L [0.14, 0.48]; I^2 = 77.2%). Montelukast was used as the comparator in two RCTs, including 317 participants. The result indicated that CHM plus montelukast was superior to montelukast alone, and the heterogeneity was 'low' (MD: 0.63 L [0.57, 0.68]; I^2 = 0.0%).

Lung Function: Peak Expiratory Flow

Thirty-seven of the 166 studies, including 2,915 participants, assessed PEF. Thirteen studies reported PEF% and 24 reported PEF litres/second (L/S). Overall meta-analyses for PEF were performed at the end of treatment based on different comparators.

Chinese Herbal Medicine versus Pharmacotherapy

Fifteen RCTs (n = 1,151) compared CHM with pharmacotherapy. Treatment duration ranged from one to eight weeks. The overall result showed no difference between CHM and pharmacotherapy (MD: 3.31% [–4.18, 10.80]; I^2 = 96.4%; MD 0.13 L/S [–0.13, 0.40]; I^2 = 50.8%) (Tables 5.14 and 5.15).

Subgroup analysis

There was no difference between CHM and pharmacotherapy in terms of PEF% or L/S when studies were subgrouped by 'low' risk of

Table 5.14. Chinese Herbal Medicine versus Pharmacotherapy: Peak Expiratory Flow (Percentage)

Descriptor	No. of Studies (Participants)	Effect Size (MD [95% CI], I^2)	Included Studies
PEF%	7 (512)	3.31 [–4.18, 10.80], 96.4%	H38, H63, H68, H86, H94, H132, H145
'Low' risk of bias: Sequence generation	5 (402)	0.72 [–8.24, 9.70], 96.6%	H63, H86, H94, H132, H145
Treatment duration: ≤ 4 weeks	6 (420)	2.61 [–5.97, 11.20], 96.8%	H38, H63, H68, H86, H94, H132
Comparator: ICS plus bronchodilators	2 (152)	8.50 [6.28, 10.73]*, 0.0%	H68, H145
Comparator: ICS plus other pharmacotherapies for PEF%	3 (252)	5.20 [0.04, 10.37]*, 61.6%	H68, H94, H145

*Statistically significant; see Chapter 4.
Abbreviations: CI, confidence interval; ICS, inhaled corticosteroids; MD, mean difference; PEF, peak expiratory flow.

Table 5.15. Chinese Herbal Medicine versus Pharmacotherapy: Peak Expiratory Flow (Litres/Second)

Descriptor	No. of Studies (Participants)	Effect Size (MD [95% CI], I^2)	Included Studies
PEF L/s	8 (639)	0.13 [–0.13, 0.40], 50.8%	H51, H110, H111, H127, H138, H144, H160, H161
'Low' risk of bias: Sequence generation	4 (321)	–0.03 [–0.20, 0.13], 0.0%	H110, H144, H160, H161
Treatment duration: ≤ four weeks	7 (579)	0.17 [–0.11, 0.45], 54.7%	H51, H110, H111, H127, H138, H144, H160
Syndrome classification: Severe wind invading the Lungs	2 (124)	0.16 [–0.76, 1.10], 68.7%	H51, H160
Comparator: ICS plus bronchodilators	4 (378)	–0.12 [–0.39, 0.15], 0.0%	H111, H144, H160, H161
Comparator: ICS plus other pharmacotherapies	5 (439)	–0.03 [–0.19, 0.12], 0.0%	H110, H111, H144, H160, H161

Abbreviations: CI, confidence interval; ICS, inhaled corticosteroids; MD, mean difference; PEF, peak expiratory flow.

bias for sequence generation, treatment duration or syndrome classification (Tables 5.14 and 5.15).

Subgroup analysis by drug class showed that PEF% was increased in the CHM groups more than those using ICS plus bronchodilators and heterogeneity was 'low' (MD: 8.50% [6.28, 10.73]; I^2 = 0.0%). However, there was no difference between CHM and ICS plus bronchodilators in terms of PEF L/S (MD: –0.12 L/S [–0.39, 0.15]; I^2 = 0.0%). Studies of ICS plus other pharmacotherapies showed a similar result. Peak expiratory flow % improved in the CHM groups more than the control group (MD: 5.20% [0.04, 10.37]; I^2 = 61.6%) but there was no difference between groups in terms of PEF L/S (MD: –0.03 L/S [–0.19, 0.12]; I^2 = 0.0%). Heterogeneity was reduced in all subgroups of comparator type.

Chinese Herbal Medicine plus Pharmacotherapy versus Pharmacotherapy Alone

Twenty-two RCTs (*n* = 1,766) compared CHM plus pharmacotherapy with pharmacotherapy alone. Treatment duration ranged from two to eight weeks. The overall result indicated that PEF% increased in participants receiving CHM plus pharmacotherapy, compared to pharmacotherapy alone, although heterogeneity was 'high' (MD: 6.85% [4.99, 8.71]; I^2 = 68.3%). The effect was also seen in PEF L/S (MD: 0.73 L/S [0.41, 1.04]; I^2 = 79.8%) (Tables 5.16 and 5.17).

Table 5.16. Chinese Herbal Medicine plus Pharmacotherapy versus Pharmacotherapy: Peak Expiratory Flow (Percentage)

Descriptor	No. of Studies (Participants)	Effect Size (MD [95% CI], I^2)	Included Studies
PEF%	5 (392)	6.85 [4.99, 8.71]*, 68.3%	H11, H17, H33, H77, H143
'Low' risk of bias: Sequence generation	2 (172)	8.62 [6.86, 10.38]*, 0.0%	H17, H143
Treatment duration: ≤ four weeks	2 (120)	6.64 [3.22, 10.06]*, 64.8%	H11, H33
Treatment duration: > four weeks	3 (272)	6.96 [4.13, 9.80]*, 78.3%	H17, H77, H143
Syndrome classification: Liver fire attacking the Lungs	2 (152)	6.95 [2.85, 11.06]*, 76.3%	H17, H33
Comparator: ICS plus bronchodilators	2 (192)	6.97 [3.56, 10.38]*, 89.1%	H17, H77
Comparator: ICS plus other pharmacotherapies	3 (252)	7.30 [4.97, 9.63]*, 82.2%	H11, H17, H77
Comparator: Montelukast	2 (124)	0.66 [0.00, 1.32], 59.2%	H5, H34

*Statistically significant; see Chapter 4.
Abbreviations: CI, confidence interval; ICS, inhaled corticosteroids; MD, mean difference; PEF, peak expiratory flow.

Table 5.17. Chinese Herbal Medicine plus Pharmacotherapy versus Pharmacotherapy: Peak Expiratory Flow (Litres/Second)

Descriptor	No. of Studies (Participants)	Effect Size (MD [95% CI], I²)	Included Studies
PEF L/S	17 (1,374)	0.73 [0.41, 1.04]*, 79.8%)	H3, H5, H6, H23, H25, H29, H34, H54, H91, H96, H119, H136, H150, H154, H156, H160, H161
'Low' risk of bias: Sequence generation	5 (344)	0.29 [–0.33, 0.92], 76.5%	H3, H5, H150, H156, H160
Treatment duration: ≤ four weeks	11 (822)	0.84 [0.38, 1.30]*, 85.7%	H3, H5, H6, H23, H25, H29, H34, H91, H119, H150, H156
Treatment duration: > four weeks	6 (552)	0.57 [0.30, 0.85]*, 15.6%	H54, H96, H136, H154, H160, H161
Syndrome classification: Severe wind attacking the Lungs	2 (170)	0.61 [–0.86, 2.10], 85.9%	H23, H156
Syndrome classification: Wind-phlegm obstructing the Lungs	2 (94)	0.30 [–0.54, 1.15], 57.3%	H6, H54
Formula: Su huang zhi ke fang 苏黄止咳方	4 (315)	1.33 [0.62, 2.04]*, 80.4%	H29, H91, H150, H154
Formula: Zhi sou san 止嗽散	3 (418)	0.84 [0.45, 1.23]*, 54.0%	H96, H119, H136
Comparator: ICS	2 (114)	1.27 [–0.89, 3.43], 93.2%	H29, H164
Comparator: ICS plus bronchodilators	6 (586)	0.46 [–0.02, 0.95], 70.8%	H6, H136, H150, H156, H160, H161
Comparator: ICS plus other pharmacotherapies	11 (999)	0.55 [0.19, 0.90]*, 76.2%	H3, H6, H23, H91, H96, H119, H136, H150, H156, H160, H161
Comparator: Montelukast	2 (124)	0.66 [0.00, 1.32], 59.2%	H5, H34

*Statistically significant; see Chapter 4.

Abbreviations: CI, confidence interval; ICS, inhaled corticosteroids; MD, mean difference; PEF, peak expiratory flow.

Subgroup analysis

Peak expiratory flow % was assessed in two studies (n = 172) that were judged at 'low' risk of bias for sequence generation. Integrative medicine was superior to pharmacotherapy, and heterogeneity was 'low' (MD: 8.62% [6.86, 10.38]; I^2 = 0.0%). Five studies (n = 344) that were judged at 'low' risk of bias for sequence generation reported PEF L/S; there was no difference between groups (MD: 0.29 L/S [–0.33, 0.92]; I^2 = 76.5%).

Treatment duration for four weeks or less in two studies (n = 120) evaluating PEF% favoured CHM plus pharmacotherapy, compared with pharmacotherapy alone, and heterogeneity remained high (MD: 6.64% [3.22, 10.06]; I^2 = 64.8%). Three RCTs including 272 participants, with treatment duration longer than four weeks, also showed CHM plus pharmacotherapy was superior to pharmaco-therapy alone (MD: 6.96% [4.13, 9.80]; I^2 = 78.3%) although heterogeneity did not decrease significantly. Treatment duration for four weeks or less in 11 studies (n = 822) assessing PEF L/S favoured CHM plus pharmacotherapy, compared to pharmacotherapy alone (MD: 0.84 L/S [0.38, 1.30]; I^2 = 85.7%). Six RCTs including 552 participants, with treatment duration longer than four weeks, showed CHM plus pharmacotherapy was better than pharmaco-therapy alone, and heterogeneity was 'low' (MD: 0.57 L/S [0.30, 0.85]; I^2 = 15.6%).

Syndrome classification of Liver fire attacking the Lungs was assessed in two studies and integrative medicine was superior to pharmacotherapy alone, although heterogeneity was substantial (MD: 6.95% [2.85, 11.06]; I^2 = 76.3%). The pooled results of the studies assessing wind-phlegm obstructing the Lungs and severe wind attacking the Lungs showed no difference between the two groups (MD: 0.30 L/S [–0.54, 1.15]; I^2 = 57.3% and MD: 0.61 L/S [–0.86, 2.10]; I^2 = 85.9%, respectively). The formulas *Su huang zhi ke fang* 苏黄止咳方 and *Zhi sou san* 止嗽散 were used in multiple studies. When combined with pharmacotherpies, both formulas were superior to pharmacotherapies alone (MD: 1.33 L/S [0.62, 2.04]; I^2 = 80.4%; and MD: 0.84 L/S [0.45, 1.23]; I^2 = 54.0%, respectively).

Subgroup analysis by drug class showed that integrative medicine was superior to ICS plus bronchodilators and ICS plus other pharmacotherapies, in terms of PEF%. There was no difference in PEF L/S, except when integrative medicine was compared to ICS plus other pharmacotherapies (MD: 0.55 L/S [0.19, 0.90]; I^2 = 76.2%); however, heterogeneity remained 'high'.

Exhaled Nitric Oxide

Four of the 166 studies, which included 274 participants, assessed FeNO. Overall meta-analyses for FeNO were performed at the end of treatment based on different comparators.

Chinese Herbal Medicine versus Pharmacotherapy

Three RCTs (*n* = 184) compared CHM with pharmacotherapy. Treatment duration ranged from four to 12 weeks. Exhaled nitric oxide was reduced (indicating improvement) in participants receiving CHM compared to pharmacotherapies, and heterogeneity was 'low' (MD: –7.50 parts per billion (ppb) [–10.10, –4.90]; I^2 = 23.1%) (Table 5.18).

Table 5.18. Chinese Herbal Medicine versus Pharmacotherapy: Exhaled Nitric Oxide

Descriptor	No. of Studies (Participants)	Effect Size (MD [95% CI], I^2)	Included Studies
FeNO ppb	3 (184)	–7.50 [–10.10, –4.90]*, 23.1%	H129, H139, H163
'Low' risk of bias: Sequence generation	2 (120)	–3.47 [–14.02, 7.07], 43.0%	H129, H163
Treatment duration: ≤ four weeks; wind-phlegm obstructing the Lungs	2 (124)	–4.13 [–16.18, 7.92], 57.7%	H129, H139

*Statistically significant; see Chapter 4.

Abbreviations: CI, confidence interval; FeNO, fractional exhaled nitric oxide; MD, mean difference.

Subgroup analysis

Subgroup analysis of two studies (*n* = 120) that were judged at 'low' risk of bias for sequence generation was performed. The result indicated that there was no difference between CHM and pharmacotherapy (MD: –3.47 ppb [–14.02, 7.07]; I^2 = 43.0%). Treatment duration of four weeks or less was reported in two studies (*n* = 124). The same two studies also included participants with a syndrome differentiation of wind-phlegm obstructing the Lungs. The results showed that there was no difference between CHM and pharmacotherapy (MD: –4.13 ppb [–16.18, 7.92]; I^2 = 57.7%).

Chinese Herbal Medicine plus Pharmacotherapy versus Pharmacotherapy

One RCT (*n* = 90) compared CHM plus pharmacotherapy with pharmacotherapy alone. Treatment duration was two weeks. The result indicated that integrative medicine was superior to pharmacotherapy alone (MD: –2.93 ppb [–6.14, –0.28]).

Eosinophil Cationic Protein

Six of the 166 studies, including 693 participants, assessed ECP. Overall meta-analyses for ECP were performed at the end of treatment based on different comparators.

Chinese Herbal Medicine versus Pharmacotherapy

Four RCTs (*n* = 501) compared CHM with pharmacotherapy. Treatment duration ranged from four to eight weeks. Meta-analysis showed that ECP was reduced (indicating improvement) in the CHM group compared to pharmacotherapy, but heterogeneity was 'high' (MD: –10.09 μg/L [–15.68, –4.50]; I^2 = 88.8%) (Table 5.19). Subgroup analysis of two studies that were judged at 'low' risk of bias for sequence generation was performed. The pooled result indicated that there was no difference between CHM and pharmacotherapy (MD: –8.72 μg/L [–19.36, 1.91]; I^2 = 92.2%). Treatment duration of four

Table 5.19. Eosinophil Cationic Protein

Descriptor	No. of Studies (Participants)	Effect Size (MD [95% CI], I^2)	Included Studies
Chinese Herbal Medicine versus Pharmacotherapy			
All studies	4 (501)	−10.09 [−15.68, −4.50], 88.8%	H46, H66, H69, H142
'Low' risk of bias: Sequence generation	2 (154)	−8.72 [−19.36, 1.91], 92.2%	H46, H142
Treatment duration: ≤ four weeks	3 (311)	−11.15 [−19.97, −2.34]*, 92.5%	H46, H69, H142
Chinese Herbal Medicine plus Pharmacotherapy versus Pharmacotherapy Alone			
All studies	2 (192)	−14.73 [−17.76, −11.70]*, 0.0%	H118, H136

*Statistically significant; see Chapter 4.
Abbreviations: CI, confidence interval; MD, mean difference.

weeks or less was reported in three studies; the result showed that CHM was better than pharmacotherapy, although heterogeneity remained 'high' (MD: −11.15 μg/L [−19.97, −2.34], $I^2 = 92.5\%$).

Chinese Herbal Medicine plus Pharmacotherapy versus Pharmacotherapy Alone

Two RCTs compared CHM plus pharmacotherapy with pharmacotherapy alone. The overall result indicated that participants receiving CHM plus pharmacotherapy were better than pharmacotherapy alone, and heterogeneity was 'low' (MD: −14.73 μg/L [−17.76, −11.70]; $I^2 = 0.0\%$) (Table 5.19).

Blood Eosinophil Count

Forty-one of the 166 studies, which included 3,265 participants, assessed EOS. Three studies reported EOS%, and 17 reported EOS $\times 10^9$/L.

Overall meta-analyses for EOS was performed at the end of treatment based on different comparators.

Chinese Herbal Medicine versus Pharmacotherapy

Twenty RCTs (n = 1,696) compared CHM with pharmacotherapy. Treatment duration ranged from two to 14 weeks. In terms of EOS%, the overall result indicated that there was no difference between CHM and pharmacotherapy (MD: –0.74% [–1.88, 0.39]; I^2 = 48.6%). Results of EOS $\times 10^9$/L also showed no difference between groups (MD: –0.02 $\times 10^9$/L [–0.06, 0.02]; I^2 = 85.7%) (Table 5.20).

Subgroup analysis

Subgrouping was only possible for studies that reported EOS $\times 10^9$/L because EOS% was only used in three studies. Subgrouping by 'low' risk of bias for sequence generation showed no difference between CHM and pharmacotherapy (MD: –0.00 $\times 10^9$/L [–0.09, 0.07]; I^2 = 91.4%, ten studies) (Table 5.20). Treatment duration of four weeks or less was reported in 12 studies (n = 1,008) and there was no difference between CHM and pharmacotherapy (MD: –0.01 $\times 10^9$/L [–0.07, 0.05]; I^2 = 90.0%). Five studies reported treatment duration of more than four weeks; the results showed CHM was not superior to pharmacotherapy (MD: –0.02b $\times 10^9$/L [–0.06, 0.02]; I^2 = 0.0%).

Four studies included participants with the syndrome classification of severe wind attacking the Lungs; meta-analysis showed no difference between groups (MD: 0.00 $\times 10^9$/L [–0.28, 0.29]; I^2 = 94.8%). The formula *Su huang zhi ke fang* 苏黄止咳方 was assesssed in four studies and the results were pooled; however, there was no difference between CHM and pharmacotherapy in terms of EOS (MD: 0.02 $\times 10^9$/L [–0.18, 0.23]; I^2 = 96.8%). Subgrouping by drug class, such as ICS plus bronchodilators, ICS plus other pharmacotherapies, or montelukast showed no difference between groups and heterogeneity remained 'high' (Table 5.20).

Table 5.20.   Chinese Herbal Medicine versus Pharmacotherapy: Blood Eosinophil Count

Descriptor	No. of Studies (Participants)	Effect Size (MD [95% CI], I^2)	Included Studies
All studies %	3 (181)	−0.74% [−1.88, 0.39], 48.6%	H95, H102, H129
All studies ×10⁹/L	17 (1,515)	−0.02 ×10⁹/L [−0.06, 0.02], 85.7%	H30, H39, H40, H47, H55, H60, H66, H69, H88, H112, H124, H130, H132, H133, H142, H160, H161
'Low' risk of bias: Sequence generation	10 (806)	−0.00 ×10⁹/L [−0.09, 0.07], 91.4%	H30, H40, H60, H124, H130, H132, H133, H142, H160, H161
Treatment duration: ≤ four weeks	12 (1,008)	−0.01 ×10⁹/L [−0.07, 0.05], 90.0%	H30, H40, H47, H55, H60, H69, H88, H112, H130, H132, H142, H160
Treatment duration: > four weeks	5 (507)	−0.02 ×10⁹/L [−0.06, 0.02], 0.0%	H39, H66, H124, H133, H161
Syndrome classification: Severe wind attacking the Lungs	4 (282)	0.00 ×10⁹/L [−0.28, 0.29], 94.8%	H30, H47, H60, H160
Formula: Su huang zhi ke fang	4 (322)	0.02 ×10⁹/L [−0.18, 0.23], 96.8%	H30, H47, H55, H60
Comparator: ICS plus bronchodilators	9 (721)	−0.01 ×10⁹/L [−0.11, 0.08], 92.3%	H30, H47, H60, H88, H124, H130, H133, H160, H161
Comparator: ICS plus other pharmacotherapies	11 (998)	−0.01 ×10⁹/L [−0.08, 0.05], 90.6%	H30, H47, H55, H60, H69, H88, H124, H130, H133, H160, H161,
Comparator: montelukast	2 (120)	−1.00% [−3.07, 1.06], 71.4%	H95, H129

Abbreviations: CI, confidence interval; MD, mean difference.

Chinese Herbal Medicine plus Pharmacotherapy versus Pharmacotherapy Alone

Twenty-three RCTs (*n* = 1,709) compared CHM plus pharmacotherapy with pharmacotherapy alone. Treatment duration ranged from ten days to eight weeks. In terms of EOS%, the overall result indicated that CHM plus pharmacotherapy was better than pharmacotherapy alone. However, heterogeneity was 'high' (MD: –2.95% [–3.77, –2.14]; I^2 = 86.7%). In terms of EOS ×10^9/L, the overall result indicated that CHM plus pharmacotherapy was superior to pharmacotherapy alone, but heterogeneity was 'high' (MD: –0.02 ×10^9/L [–0.05, –0.00]; I^2 = 60.5%) (Table 5.21).

Table 5.21. Chinese Herbal Medicine plus Pharmacotherapy versus Pharmacotherapy Alone: Blood Eosinophil Count

Descriptor	No. of Studies (Participants)	Effect Size (MD [95% CI], I^2)	Included Studies
All studies	6 (558)	–2.95% [–3.77, –2.14]*, 86.7%	H25, H49, H65, H84, H100, H155
	17 (1,151)	–0.02 ×10^9/L [–0.05, –0.00]*, 60.5%	H3, H11, H16, H21, H22, H33, H43, H57, H61, H82, H91, H118, H136, H143, H149, H160, H161
'Low' risk of bias: Sequence generation	2 (186)	–3.45% [–5.61, –1.31]*, 93.1%	H65, H100
	9 (530)	0.03 ×10^9/L [–0.06, 0.00], 38.1%	H3, H21, H43, H57, H61, H143, H149, H160, H161
Treatment duration: ≤ four weeks	5 (462)	–2.66% [–3.43, –1.89]*, 83.0%	H25, H49, H84, H100, H155
	13 (874)	–0.02 ×10^9/L [–0.05, 0.00], 67.5%	H3, H11, H21, H22, H33, H43, H57, H61, H82, H118, H136, H149, H160

(Continued)

Table 5.21. (*Continued*)

Descriptor	No. of Studies (Participants)	Effect Size (MD [95% CI], I^2)	Included Studies
Treatment duration: > four weeks	4 (277)	0.04 ×10⁹/L [−0.10, 0.01], 0.0%	H16, H91, H143, H161
Syndrome classification: Severe wind attacking the Lungs	5 (306)	−0.00 ×10⁹/L [−0.03, 0.03], 52.0%	H43, H61, H82, H118, H160
Syndrome classification: Liver fire attacking the Lungs	2 (100)	−0.04 ×10⁹/L [−0.311, 0.23], 0.0%	H3, H33
Syndrome classification: Phlegm-dampness obstructing the Lungs	2 (120)	−0.05 ×10⁹/L [−0.07, −0.02]*, 0.0%	H21, H57
Formula: Su huang zhi ke fang 苏黄止咳方	4 (396)	−2.97% [−3.78, −2.16]*, 83.2%	H49, H84, H100, H155
	2 (140)	−0.14 ×10⁹/L [−0.42, 0.14], 65.7%	H43, H143
Comparator: ICS plus bronchodilators	4 (386)	0.00% [−0.06, 0.06], 0.0%	H65, H84, H100, H155
	8 (602)	0.01 ×10⁹/L [−0.04, 0.01], 65.8%	H16, H22, H61, H82, H136, H149, H160, H161
Comparator: ICS plus other pharmacotherapies	4 (386)	−3.14% [−4.12, −2.15]*, 84.5%	H65, H84, H100, H155
	12 (819)	−0.02 ×10⁹/L [−0.05, 0.00], 64.1%	H3, H11, H16, H22, H43, H61, H82, H91, H136, H149, H160, H161

*Statistically significant; see Chapter 4.
Abbreviations: CI, confidence interval; ICS, inhaled corticosteroids; MD, mean difference.

Subgroup analysis

In terms of studies at 'low' risk of bias for sequence generation, two measured EOS% and integrative medicine was superior to control groups, but heterogeneity remained 'high' (MD: −3.45% [−5.61, −1.31], I^2 = 93.1%). Nine studies at 'low' risk of bias for sequence generation measured EOS ×10^9/L but there was no difference between groups and heterogeneity remained high (MD: 0.03 ×10^9/L [−0.06, 0.00], I^2 = 38.1%) (Table 5.21). Treatment duration for four weeks or less was assessed in five studies (n = 462) with EOS (%) favouring CHM plus pharmacotherapy, compared with pharmacotherapy alone (MD: −2.66% [−3.43, −1.89]; I^2 = 83.0%). One RCT (H65) including 96 participants, with treatment duration longer than four weeks, showed CHM plus pharmacotherapy was better than pharmacotherapy alone (MD: −4.63% [−5.75, −3.50]).

Treatment duration of four weeks or less was reported in five studies measuring EOS% and integrative medicine was superior to control groups, but heterogeneity remained 'high' (MD: −2.66% [−3.43, −1.89], I^2 = 83.0%). Eosinophils ×10^9/L was also subgrouped by treatment duration but CHM plus pharmacotherapy was not superior to pharmacotherapy alone, although heterogeneity was reduced (Table 5.21). Heterogeneity was also reduced when studies were subgrouped by syndrome classification, but the meta-analysis results showed no difference between groups, except for two studies assessing phlegm-dampness obstructing the Lungs (MD: −0.05 ×10^9/L [−0.07, −0.02]; I^2 = 0.0%).

Su huang zhi ke fang 苏黄止咳方 was the only formula that could be subgrouped. Results of EOS% showed that integrative medicine was superior to control groups, but heterogeneity remained 'high' (MD: −2.97% [−3.78, −2.16]; I^2 = 83.2%). There was no difference between groups when *Su huang zhi ke fang* 苏黄止咳方 was subgrouped by EOS ×10^9/L (MD: −0.14 ×10^9/L [−0.42, 0.14]; I^2 = 65.7%). Subgrouping by drug class did not show significant differences between groups, except for ICS plus other pharmacotherapies in four studies evaluating EOS%, but heterogeneity remained 'high' (MD: −3.14% [−4.12, −2.15]; I^2 = 84.5%) (Table 5.21).

Cough Reflex Sensitivity

One of the 166 studies assessed cough reflex sensitivity. The study included 161 participants with Lung *yin* deficiency and compared CHM formula *Min ke jian* 敏咳煎 to a bronchodilator for four weeks. In terms of cough reflex sensitivity C2 and C5, the result indicated that CHM was superior to bronchodilators (MD: 0.72 [0.58, 0.85]) and (MD: 0.21 [0.05, 0.36]), respectively.

Total Effective Rate

One hundred and fifty-two of the 166 studies, including 12,873 participants, assessed total effective rate. Effective rate was classified as the number of people with improved symptoms and signs. Treatments were classified as effective in people with clinically controlled, or markedly improved, symptoms, and treatments were considered ineffective when people only reported a limited improvement or no symptom improvement. Meta-analyses for total effective rate were performed at the end of treatment based on different comparators using risk ratio (RR) and 95% confidence intervals (CI) (see Chapter 4 for details).

Chinese Herbal Medicine versus Placebo

One RCT, with 72 participants, compared CHM formula *Qu feng xuan fei fang* 祛风宣肺方 with placebo. The result showed CHM was superior to placebo (RR: 2.86 [1.42, 5.73]).

Chinese Herbal Medicine versus Pharmacotherapy

Eighty RCTs (*n* = 6,642) compared CHM with pharmacotherapy. Treatment duration ranged from one to 12 weeks. The overall result showed an improvement in the CHM group compared to the pharmacotherapy group (RR: 1.33 [1.26, 1.40]; I^2 = 56.4%) (Table 5.22).

Subgroup analysis

Subgroup analysis of 36 studies that were judged at 'low' risk of bias for sequence generation showed a similar result as the overall pool

Table 5.22. Chinese Herbal Medicine versus Pharmacotherapy: Total Effective Rate

Descriptor	No. of Studies (Participants)	Effect Size (RR [95% CI], I^2)	Included Studies
All studies	80 (6,642)	1.33 [1.26, 1.40]*, 56.4%	H1, H4, H7–H9, H18–H20, H24, H30–H32, H35, H38–H40, H45, H47, H48, H51, H53, H55, H60, H62, H63, H66, H68, H69–H73, H75, H76, H78–H81, H83, H86, H87, H89, H90, H94, H95, H98, H102–H104, H109–H113, H115, H117, H120, H123, H124, H127, H129, H130–H133, H138–H142, H144–H147, H152, H153, H157, H160, H161, H163
'Low' risk of bias: Sequence generation	36 (2925)	1.33 [1.23, 1.44]*, 53.6%	H1, H7, H18, H20, H30, H32, H40, H48, H60, H62, H63, H72, H73, H75, H78, H81, H86, H94, H95, H102, H103, H110, H115, H120, H124, H129, H130, H132, H133, H142, H144, H145, H146, H160, H161, H163
Treatment duration: ≤ four weeks	62 (5096)	1.34 [1.27, 1.43]*, 56.3%	H1, H4, H7, H8, H18, H20, H24, H30, H32, H35, H38, H40, H45, H47, H48, H51, H55, H60, H62, H63, H68–H73, H78–H81, H86, H87, H89, H90, H94, H95, H98, H102, H103, H109–H113, H117, H120, H123, H127, H129,

Table 5.22.   (*Continued*)

Descriptor	No. of Studies (Participants)	Effect Size (RR [95% CI], I^2)	Included Studies
			H130, H132, H138–H142, H144, H146, H147, H153, H157, H160
Treatment duration: > four weeks	18 (1546)	1.28 [1.16, 1.41]*, 55.0%	H9, H19, H31, H39, H53, H66, H75, H76, H83, H104, H115, H124, H131, H133, H145, H152, H161, H163
Syndrome classification: Severe wind attacking the Lungs	17 (1145)	1.40 [1.21, 1.61]*, 61.3%	H4, H18, H19, H30, H32, H45, H47, H51, H60, H68, H73, H78, H83, H95, H115, H160, H163
Syndrome classification: Wind-phlegm obstructing the Lungs	4 (247)	1.37 [1.10, 1.70]*, 73.7%	H48, H81, H129, H139
Syndrome classification: Liver fire attacking the Lungs	3 (149)	1.17 [0.82, 1.66], 79.8%	H40, H75, H79
Syndrome classification: Hot-phlegm obstructing the Lungs	2 (152)	1.28 [1.02, 1.61]*, 0.0%	H70, H86
Syndrome classification: Phlegm-dampness obstructing the Lungs	2 (145)	1.37 [1.10, 1.70]*, 0.0%	H62, H127

(*Continued*)

Table 5.22. (Continued)

Descriptor	No. of Studies (Participants)	Effect Size (RR [95% CI], I^2)	Included Studies
Formula: *Su huang zhi ke fang* 苏黄止咳方	6 (460)	1.51 [1.15, 1.99]*, 58.1%	H30, H47, H55, H60, H89, H138
Formula: *Zhi sou san* 止嗽散	4 (309)	1.31 [1.04, 1.66]*, 47.9%	H73, H83, H103, H157
Formula: *Xiao qing long tang* 小青龙汤	3 (219)	1.37 [1.05, 1.80]*, 33.3%	H71, H90, H123
Comparator: ICS plus bronchodilators	26 (2,027)	1.29 [1.17, 1.42]*, 56.1%	H4, H8, H14, H19, H30–H32, H45, H47, H60, H68, H73, H75, H79, H81, H102, H111, H124, H130, H133, H139, H145, H152, H153, H160, H161
Comparator: ICS plus other pharmacotherapies	34 (2,742)	1.32 [1.22, 1.44]*, 55.5%	H4, H7, H8, H19, H30–32, H45, H47, H55, H60, H68, H69, H73, H75, H78, H79, H81, H94, H102, H110, H111, H113, H115, H124, H130, H133, H139, H144, H145, H152, H153, H160, H161
Comparator: Montelukast	10 (971)	1.57 [1.34, 1.84]*, 57.1%	H1, H18, H51, H72, H89, H95, H104, H120, H129, H132

*Statistically significant, see Chapter 4.
Abbreviations: CI, confidence interval; ICS, inhaled corticosteroids; RR, risk ratio.

(RR: 1.33 [1.23, 1.44]; I^2 = 53.6%). Treatment duration of four weeks or less, and longer than four weeks, showed CHM was superior to pharmacotherapy, but again the results were similar to the overall pool (Table 5.22).

The subgroup results of syndrome classification showed that participants with severe wind attacking the Lungs and hot-phlegm obstructing the Lungs who were taking CHM improved more than people taking pharmacotherapies. However, there was no difference between groups in studies assessing participants with wind-phlegm obstructing the Lungs and Liver fire attacking the Lungs. Heterogeneity was only reduced in pools that had two studies. Subgroup analysis by formula showed that *Su huang zhi ke fang* 苏黄止咳方 (six studies), *Zhi sou san* 止嗽散 (four studies) and *Xiao qing long tang* 小青龙汤 (three studies) were superior to pharmacotherapies, but results were similar to the overall pool and herterogeneity remained 'moderate'.

Subgroup analysis by drug class included comparators of ICS plus bronchodilators (26 studies), ICS plus other pharmacotherapies (34 studies) and montelukast (ten studies). All three subgroups showed that CHM was superior to the pharmacotherapies alone. The results were similar to the overall pool of studies in terms of effect and heterogeneity (Table 5.22).

Chinese Herbal Medicine plus Pharmacotherapy versus Pharmacotherapy

Seventy-three RCTs (n = 6,159) compared CHM plus pharmacotherapy with pharmacotherapy alone. Treatment duration ranged from four to 12 weeks. Chinese herbal medicine plus pharmacotherapies were superior to pharmacotherapies alone (RR: 1.33 [1.27, 1.39]; 52.7%) (Table 5.23).

Subgroup analysis

Subgroup analysis of 27 studies (n = 2,198) that were judged at 'low' risk of bias for sequence generation was performed. The pooled result was similar to the overall pool and showed that CHM plus pharmacotherapy was superior to pharmacotherapy alone, although heterogeneity remained 'high' (RR: 1.36 [1.25, 1.47]; I^2 = 55.6%). Treatment duration of four weeks or less, and duration longer than

Table 5.23. Chinese Herbal Medicine plus Pharmacotherapy versus Pharmacotherapy: Total Effective Rate

Descriptor	No. of Studies (Participants)	Effect Size (RR [95% CI], I^2)	Included Studies
All studies	73 (6,159)	1.33 [1.27, 1.39]*, 52.7%	H2, H3, H5, H6, H10–H17, H21–H23, H25–H29, H33, H36, H37, H41, H43, H44, H49, H50, H52, H54, H56, H58, H61, H64, H65, H67, H74, H77, H82, H85, H91, H92, H93, H97, H99, H100, H105–H108, H114, H116, H118, H119, H121, H122, H125, H128, H134–H137, H143, H150, H151, H154–H156, H158–H161, H165
'Low' risk of bias: Sequence generation	27 (2,198)	1.36 [1.25, 1.47]*, 55.6%	H3, H5, H10, H12, H14, H17, H21, H28, H36, H37, H43, H56, H58, H61, H65, H100, H114, H121, H125, H128, H134, H137, H143, H154, H160, H161, H165
Treatment duration: ≤ four weeks	51 (3,839)	1.35 [1.27, 1.43]*, 55.1%	H2, H3, H5, H6, H10–H15, H21–H23, H25, H27–H29, H33, H36, H41, H43, H44, H49, H50, H52, H54, H61, H64, H67, H82, H85, H93, H99, H100, H106–108, H114, H116, H118, H121, H122, H135–H137, H151, H154, H155, H158–160
Treatment duration: > four weeks	22 (2,252)	1.30 [1.20, 1.40], 50.0%	H16, H17, H26, H37, H56, H58, H65, H74, H77, H91, H92, H97, H105, H119, H125, H128, H134, H143, H150, H156, H161, H165

Table 5.23.   (*Continued*)

Descriptor	No. of Studies (Participants)	Effect Size (RR [95% CI], I²)	Included Studies
Syndrome classification: Severe wind attacking the Lungs	13 (888)	1.46 [1.24, 1.73]*, 70.1%	H10, H23, H41, H43, H50, H56, H61, H82, H99, H100, H114, H118, H160
Syndrome classification: Wind-phlegm obstructing the Lungs	5 (366)	1.24 [1.12, 1.37]*, 0.0%	H6, H14, H28, H52, H91
Syndrome classification: Liver fire attacking the Lungs	3 (192)	1.72 [1.33, 2.23]*, 0.0%	H3, H17, H33
Syndrome classification: Hot-phlegm obstructing the Lungs	3 (206)	1.30 [1.07, 1.58]*, 0.0%	H2, H85, H128
Formula: Su huang zhi ke fang 苏黄止咳方	14 (1,413)	1.34 [1.20, 1.49]*, 55.6%	H15, H29, H43, H49, H74, H97, H100, H116, H134, H143, H154–156, H159
Formula: Zhi sou san 止嗽散	5 (616)	1.22 [1.11, 1.33]*, 5.3%	H52, H106, H119, H136, H150
Formula: Xiao qing long tang 小青龙汤	3 (180)	1.04 [0.94, 1.16], 0.0%	H12, H13, H99
Comparator: ICS plus bronchodilator	29 (2,729)	1.32 [1.22, 1.42]*, 64.3%	H6, H16, H17, H22, H26, H28, H37, H50, H52, H56, H58, H61, H64, H65, H67, H74, H77, H82, H85, H100, H105, H134, H136, H150, H155, H156, H158, H160, H161

(*Continued*)

Table 5.23.   (*Continued*)

Descriptor	No. of Studies (Participants)	Effect Size (RR [95% CI], I^2)	Included Studies
Comparator: ICS plus other pharmacotherapies	44 (3,744)	1.32 [1.24, 1.40]*, 58.6%	H3, H6, H11, H13, H16, H17, H22, H23, H26, H28, H37, H41, H43, H50, H52, H56, H58, H61, H64, H65, H67, H74, H77, H82, H85, H91, H92, H100, H105, H107, H108, H119, H128, H134, H135, H136, H137, H150, H151, H155, H156, H158, H160, H161
Comparator: montelukast	9 (864)	1.32 [1.14, 1.53]*, 63.6%	H5, H12, H27, H54, H97, H99, H121, H125, H159

*Statistically significant; see Chapter 4.

Abbreviations: CI, confidence interval; ICS, inhaled corticosteroids; RR, risk ratio.

four weeks, showed integrative medicine was superior to control groups, similar to the overall pool (Table 5.23).

Four subgroups were evaluated based on syndrome classification, including severe wind attacking the Lungs, wind-phlegm obstructing the Lungs, Liver fire attacking the Lungs and hot-phlegm obstructing the Lungs. All syndrome subgroups showed that CHM plus pharmacotherapy was superior to pharmacotherapy alone. Heterogeneity was reduced in the subgroups, except for 13 studies of severe wind attacking the Lungs. Three formulas were evaluated in multiple studies and subgrouped. *Su huang zhi ke fang* 苏黄止咳方 (14 studies) and *Zhi sou san* 止嗽散 (five studies) were superior to control. Heterogeneity remained high in the *Su huang zhi ke fang* 苏黄止咳方 subgroup but not *Zhi sou san* 止嗽散 (RR: 1.22 [1.11, 1.33]; $I^2 = 5.3\%$). Results from the *Xiao qing long tang* 小青龙汤 studies showed no differnece between groups. Subgroup analysis by drug class revealed similar results to the overall pool in terms of effect size and heterogeneity.

Assessment Using Grading of Recommendations Assessment, Development and Evaluation

An assessment of the strength and quality (certainty) of the evidence from RCTs was made using Grading of Recommendations Assessment, Development and Evaluation (GRADE). Interventions, comparators and outcomes to be included were selected based on a consensus process, described in Chapter 4. Chinese herbal medicine interventions were assessed overall; GRADE tables are based on the following four comparisons:

1. CHM versus ICS and bronchodilators (Table 5.24);
2. CHM plus ICS and bronchodilators versus ICS and bronchodilators alone (Table 5.25);
3. CHM versus montelukast (Table 5.26);
4. CHM plus montelukast versus montelukast alone (Table 5.27).

Table 5.24. Chinese Herbal Medicine versus Inhaled Corticosteroids plus Bronchodilators

Outcome	Absolute Effect		Relative Effect (95% CI) No. of Participants and Studies	Certainty of the Evidence (GRADF)
	With CHM	Without CHM		
LCQ Scale from 3 to 21[a] Treatment duration: Range two to six weeks	**9.79** Average difference: 0.41 points higher (95% CI: 0.73 fewer to 1.56 more points)	**9.38**	**MD 0.41** (−0.73, 1.56) Based on data from 127 patients in two studies	⊕◯◯◯ VERY LOW[1,2,3]
Cough symptom score Treatment duration: Range four to eight weeks	—		**SMD −0.89 SD** (−0.89, 0.39) Based on data from 369 patients in five studies	⊕⊕◯◯ LOW[1,2]
FEV$_1$ Treatment duration: Range 4 to 12 weeks	**91.75** Average difference: 3.12% higher (95% CI: 1.38% higher to 4.85% higher)	**88.63**	**MD 3.12** (1.38 to 4.85) Based on data from 204 patients in three studies	⊕⊕◯◯ LOW[1,3]

(Continued)

Table 5.24. (*Continued*)

Outcome	Absolute Effect		Relative Effect (95% CI) No. of Participants and Studies	Certainty of the Evidence (GRADE)
	With CHM	Without CHM		
PEF Treatment duration: Range four to eight weeks	**89.89** Average difference: 8.5% higher (95% CI: 6.28% higher to 10.73% higher)	**81.39**	**MD 8.5** (6.28, 10.73) Based on data from 152 patients in two studies	⊕⊕◯◯ LOW[1,3]
Effective rate Treatment duration: Range one to 12 weeks	**71** per 100 Difference: 16 more per 100 patients (95% CI: 9 to 23 more per 100 patients)	**55** per 100	**RR 1.29** (1.17 to 1.42) Based on data from 2,027 patients in 26 studies	⊕⊕◯◯ LOW[1,2]
Adverse events Based on data from 1,054 patients in 14 studies	The CHM groups had a total of five AEs. The most common were nausea (two cases) and distention of the stomach (two cases). The ICS plus bronchodilator groups reported 25 AEs. The most common were hoarseness (eight cases), abnormal liver function (five cases), palpitations (three cases) and hand tremors (three cases).			

The risk in the intervention group (and its 95% confidence interval) is based on the assumed risk in the comparison group and the relative effect of the intervention (and its 95% CI).

Abbreviations: AE, adverse event; CHM, Chinese herbal medicine; CI, confidence interval; FEV_1, forced expiratory volume-one second; LCQ, Leicester cough questionnaire; MD, mean difference; PEF, peak expiratory flow; RR, risk ratio; SMD, standardised mean difference.

Notes
[a]Higher scores indicate less symptoms:
[1]Unclear sequence generation and allocation concealment; lack of blinding of participants and personnel.
[2]Considerable statistical heterogeneity.
[3]Small sample size.

Study references
LCQ: H75, H102
Cough symptom score: H19, H124, H133, H162, H166
FEV_1: H88, H160, H161
PEF: H68, H145
Effective rate: H4, H8, H19, H30–H32, H45, H47, H60, H68, H73, H75, H79, H81, H102, H111, H124, H130, H133, H139, H144, H145, H152, H153, H160, H161
Adverse events: H8, H19, H30, H47, H60, H68, H81, H88, H102, H133, H144, H160–162, H166

Table 5.25. Chinese Herbal Medicine plus Inhaled Corticosteroids plus Bronchodilators versus Inhaled Corticosteroids plus Bronchodilators Alone

Outcome	Absolute Effect		Relative Effect (95% CI) No. of Participants and Studies	Certainty of the Evidence (GRADE)
	With CHM	**Without CHM**		
LCQ Scale from 3 to 21[a] Treatment duration: ten days	**18.07** Average difference: 2.66 points higher (95% CI: 2.15 to 3.16 more points)	**15.41**	**MD 2.66** (2.15, 3.16) Based on data from 88 patients in one study	⊕⊕○○ LOW[1,2]
Cough symptom score Treatment duration: Range ten days to eight weeks	—		**SMD –1.24 SD** (–1.76, –0.73) Based on data from 394 patients in six studies	⊕⊕○○ LOW[1,3]
FEV$_1$ Treatment duration: Range four to 12 weeks	**94.95** Average difference: 8.79% higher (95% CI: 7.44% higher to 10.14% higher)	**86.16**	**MD 8.79** (7.44 to 10.14) Based on data from 300 patients in four studies	⊕⊕○○ LOW[1,2]
PEF Treatment duration: Mean one month	**90.95** Average difference: 6.97% higher (95% CI: 3.56% higher to 10.38% higher)	**83.98**	**MD 6.97** (3.56, 10.38) Based on data from 192 patients in two studies	⊕○○○ VERY LOW[1,2,3]
Effective rate Treatment duration: Range one to 12 weeks	**82** per 100 Difference: 20 more per 100 patients (95% CI: 14 to 26 more per 100 patients)	**62** per 100	**RR 1.32** (1.22 to 1.42) Based on data from 2,729 patients in 29 studies	⊕⊕○○ LOW[1,3]
Adverse events Based on data from 1,854 patients in 23 studies	The integrative CHM group had a total of 26 AEs; the most common were nausea (five cases), vomiting (five cases) and dental ulcer (four cases). The ICS plus bronchodilator groups reported 51 AEs; the most common were nausea (14 cases), palpitation (seven cases), dental ulcer (seven cases), dry mouth (four cases) and dizziness (four cases).			

(Continued)

Table 5.25.   (*Continued*)

The risk in the intervention group (and its 95% confidence interval) is based on the assumed risk in the comparison group and the relative effect of the intervention (and its 95% CI). Abbreviations: AE, adverse event; CHM, Chinese herbal medicine; CI, confidence interval; FEV$_1$, forced expiratory volume-one second; LCQ, Leicester cough questionnaire; MD, mean difference; PEF, peak expiratory flow; RR, risk ratio; SMD, standardised mean difference.

Notes

[a]Higher scores indicate less symptoms.

[1]Unclear sequence generation and allocation concealment; lack of blinding of participants and personnel.

[2]Small sample size.

[3]Considerable statistical heterogeneity.

Study references

LCQ: H149

Cough symptom score: H16, H28, H56, H149, H162, H166

FEV$_1$: H28, H77, H160, H161

PEF: H17, H77

Effective rate: H6, H16–17, H22, H26, H28, H37, H50, H52, H56, H58, H61, H64, H65, H67, H74, H77, H82, H85, H100, H105, H134, H136, H150, H155, H156, H158, H160, H161

Adverse events: H6, H16, H28, H37, H56, H58, H61, H64, H65, H67, H82, H84, H85, H100, H105, H134, H149, H155, H156, H158, H160, H161, H166

Table 5.26.   Chinese Herbal Medicine versus Montelukast

Outcome	Absolute Effect		Relative Effect (95% CI) No. of Participants and Studies	Certainty of the Evidence (GRADE)
	With CHM	Without CHM		
LCQ Scale from 3 to 21[a] Treatment duration: Range two to four weeks	**15.30** Average difference: 2.23 points higher (95% CI: 0.81 to 3.65 more points)	**13.07**	**MD 2.23** (0.81, 3.65) Based on data from 345 patients in five studies	⊕◯◯◯ VERY LOW[1,2,3]
Cough symptom score Treatment duration: Range two to eight weeks	—		**SMD –0.79 SD** (–1.08, –0.51) Based on data from 454 patients in six studies	⊕⊕◯◯ LOW[1,2]
FEV$_1$ Treatment duration: two weeks	**90.67** Average difference: 2.84% higher (95% CI: 0.34% higher to 5.33% higher)	**87.83**	**MD 2.84** (0.34 to 5.33) Based on data from 48 patients in one study	⊕⊕◯◯ LOW[1,3]

(Continued)

Table 5.26. (*Continued*)

Outcome	Absolute Effect		Relative Effect (95% CI) No. of Participants and Studies	Certainty of the Evidence (GRADE)
	With CHM	Without CHM		
PEF Treatment duration: two weeks	89.04 Average difference: 3.91% higher (95% CI: 0.90% higher to 6.91% higher)	85.13	MD 3.91 (0.90, 6.91) Based on data from 48 patients in one study	⊕⊕○○ LOW[1,3]
Effective rate Treatment duration: Range ten days to eight weeks	78 per 100 Difference: 28 more per 100 patients (95% CI: 17 to 42 more per 100 patients)	50 per 100	RR 1.57 (1.34 to 1.84) Based on data from 971 patients in ten studies	⊕⊕○○ LOW[1,2]
Adverse events Based on data from 286 patients in four studies	Two AEs of constipation occurred in the CHM group. The montelukast groups reported four AEs, including diarrhoea (two cases) and nausea (two cases).			

The risk in the intervention group (and its 95% confidence interval) is based on the assumed risk in the comparison group and the relative effect of the intervention (and its 95% CI).

Abbreviations: AE, adverse event; CHM, Chinese herbal medicine; CI, confidence interval; FEV_1, forced expiratory volume-one second; LCQ, Leicester cough questionnaire; MD, mean difference; PEF, peak expiratory flow; RR, risk ratio; SMD, standardised mean difference.

Notes

[a]Higher scores indicate less symptoms.

[1]Unclear sequence generation and allocation concealment; lack of blinding of participants and personnel.

[2]Considerable statistical heterogeneity.

[3]Small sample size.

Study references

LCQ: H18, H72, H120, H126, H129

Cough symptom score: H72, H89, H95, H104, H120, H132

FEV1: H132

PEF: H132

Effective rate: H1, H18, H51, H72, H89, H95, H104, H120, H129, H132

Adverse events: H89, H104, H129, H132

Table 5.27.   Chinese Herbal Medicine plus Montelukast versus Montelukast Alone

Outcome	Absolute Effect		Relative Effect (95% CI) No. of Participants and Studies	Certainty of the Evidence (GRADE)
	With CHM	Without CHM		
LCQ – not reported				
Cough symptom score Scale from: 0 to 12[a] Treatment duration: 14 days	1.21 Average difference: 1.15 points lower (95% CI: 1.27 to 1.02 fewer points)	2.36	MD –1.15 (–1.27 to –1.02) Based on data from 84 patients in one study	⊕⊕○○ LOW[1,2]
FEV$_1$ Treatment duration: two weeks	83.51 Average difference: 4.39% higher (95% CI: 1.24% lower to 10.02% higher)	79.12	MD 4.39 (–1.24 to 10.02) Based on data from 36 patients in one study	⊕⊕○○ LOW[1,3]
PEF – not reported				
Effective rate Treatment duration: Range two weeks to one month	74 per 100 Difference: 18 more per 100 patients (95% CI: 8 to 30 more per 100 patients)	56 per 100	RR 1.32 (1.14 to 1.53) Based on data from 864 patients in nine studies	⊕⊕○○ LOW[1,4]
Adverse events Based on data from 279 patients in one study	Integrative CHM group had a total of six AEs, including dizziness (three cases), vomiting (two cases) and sleepiness (one case). The montelukast group reported 21 AEs; the most common were rash (six cases), dizziness (five cases) and sleepiness (five cases).			

The risk in the intervention group (and its 95% confidence interval) is based on the assumed risk in the comparison group and the relative effect of the intervention (and its 95% CI).

Abbreviations: AE, adverse event; CHM, Chinese herbal medicine; CI, confidence interval; FEV$_1$, forced expiratory volume-one second; LCQ, Leicester cough questionnaire; MD, mean difference; PEF, peak expiratory flow; RR, risk ratio.

Notes
[a] Lower scores indicate less symptoms.
[1] Unclear sequence generation and allocation concealment; lack of blinding of participants and personnel.

(Continued)

---

[2]Small sample size.
[3]Wide confidence interval and small sample size.
[4]Considerable statistical heterogeneity.

Study references
Cough symptom score: H121
FEV1: H34
Effective rate: H5, H12, H27, H54, H97, H99, H121, H125, H159
Adverse events: H97

Randomised Controlled Trial Evidence for Individual Formulas

One hundred and thirty-two named formulas and 34 unnamed formulas were reported in 166 RCTs. Evidence for the most common (top ten) individual formulas used in two or more studies are separately analysed.

Su Huang Zhi Ke Fang 苏黄止咳方

Su huang zhi ke fang 苏黄止咳方 was evaluated in 24 studies (H15, H29, H30, I143, H47, H49, H55, H60, H74, H84, H89, H96, H97, H100, H116, H134, H138, H143, H154–156, H159, H162, H166).

Cough symptom score

Su huang zhi ke fang did not significantly reduce cough symptom score, compared to pharmacotherapy, in three studies with 218 participants (MD: –0.04 points [–0.65, 0.55]; I^2 = 88.5%). Three studies (H29, H162, H166) (*n* = 202) combined *Su huang zhi ke fang* with pharmacotherapy and it was superior to pharmacotherapy alone (MD: –1.08 points [–1.78, –0.37]; I^2 = 95.6%).

Forced expiratory volume in one second

Su huang zhi ke fang improved FEV$_1$ L but there was no significant difference compared to pharmacotherapy in one study (H138) with

40 participants (MD: 0.41 L [–0.03, 0.85]). Nine studies (H29, H84, H96, H97, H100, H143, H154, H156, H159) (*n* = 953) combined *Su huang zhi ke fang* with pharmacotherapy and this was superior to pharmacotherapy alone (MD: 0.51 L [0.20, 0.82]; I^2 = 98.3%).

Peak expiratory flow

In terms of PEF %, *Su huang zhi ke fang* combined with pharmacotherapy was better than pharmacotherapy alone in one study (H138) with 80 participants (MD: 7.0% [1.04, 12.95]). In terms of PEF L/S, *Su huang zhi ke fang* was not superior to pharmacotherapy in one study with 40 participants (MD: 0.45 L/S [–0.55, 1.45]). Four studies (H29, H91, H150, H154) (*n* = 315) combined *Su huang zhi ke fang* with pharmacotherapy and it was superior to pharmacotherapy alone (MD: 1.33 L/S [0.62, 2.04]; I^2 = 80.4%).

Blood eosinophil count

Su huang zhi ke fang was not superior to pharmacotherapy in terms of reducing EOS in four studies (H30, H47, H55, H60) with 322 participants (MD: 0.02 ×10⁹/L [–0.18, 0.23]; I^2 = 96.8%). Combined with pharmacotherapy, *Su huang zhi ke fang* was superior to pharmacotherapy in four studies (H49, H84, H100, H155) with 396 participants (MD: –2.97 % [–3.78, –2.16]; I^2 = 83.2%), but not superior in terms of EOS ×10⁹/L in two studies (H43, H143) with 140 participants (MD: –0.14 ×10⁹/L [–0.42, 0.14]; I^2 = 65.7%).

Total effective rate

Su huang zhi ke fang improved total effective rate compared with pharmacotherapy alone in six studies (H30, H47, H55, H60, H89, H138) with 261 participants (RR: 1.51 [1.15, 1.99]; I^2 = 58.1%). *Su huang zhi ke fang* combined with pharmacotherapy was also superior to pharmacotherapy in 14 studies (H15, H29, H43, H49, H74, H97, H100, H116, H134, H143, H154–H156, H159) with 941 participants (RR: 1.34 [1.20, 1.49]; I^2 = 55.6%).

Adverse events

Five studies (H89, H100, H138, H155, H156) reported that no adverse events occurred in the studies. Two studies reported there were no adverse events in the treatment group, but there was one case of dental ulcer in the control group. One study reported one case of nausea in the treatment group, but there were no adverse events in the control group. One study reported mild discomfort in the throat and hoarseness of voice in both their treatment and control groups. In six integrative medicine studies (H84, H96, H97, H116, H134, H154), a total of 19 adverse events were reported in the treatment group, including dizziness (six cases), drowsiness (five cases), fatigue (three cases), vomiting (two cases), gastrointestinal discomfort (one case), dry mouth (one case) and liver dysfunction (one case). The control group reported 45 adverse events including drowsiness (14 cases), dizziness (11 cases), fatigue (seven cases), rash (six cases), nausea (two cases), dry month (three cases), liver dysfunction (one case) and mouth cavity infection (one case).

Su huang zhi ke fang 苏黄止咳方 *assessment using GRADE*

The most common formula evaluated in RCTs, *Su huang zhi ke fang*, was assessed using the GRADE approach. *Su huang zhi ke fang* was assessed compared to ICS and bronchodilators (Table 5.28), and as integrative medicine combined with ICS and bronchodilators compared to the same pharmacotherapies alone (Table 5.29).

Table 5.28.   Su huang zhi ke fang 苏黄止咳方 versus Inhaled Corticosteroids and Bronchodilators

Outcome	Absolute Effect		Relative Effect (95% CI) No. of Participants and Studies	Certainty of the Evidence (GRADE)
	With CHM	**Without CHM**		
LCQ – not reported				
Cough symptom score Scale from: 0 to 12[a] Treatment duration: Mean four weeks	**1.81** Average difference: 0.21 points higher (95% CI: 0.07 to 0.35 more points)	**1.60**	**MD 0.21** (0.07, 0.35) Based on data from 120 patients in two studies	⊕⊕◯◯ LOW[1,2]
FEV$_1$ – not reported				
PEF – not reported				
Effective rate Treatment duration: Mean four weeks	**58** per 100 Difference: 7 more per 100 patients (95% CI: 6 fewer to 21 more per 100 patients)	**51** per 100	**RR 1.13** (0.89 to 1.42) Based on data from 202 patients in three studies	⊕⊕◯◯ LOW[1,2]
Adverse events Based on data from 263 patients in four studies	Only one AE of nausea occurred in the *Su huang zhi ke fang* 苏黄止咳方 group. The ICS plus bronchodilator groups reported six AEs, including hoarseness (four cases) and dental ulcer (two cases).			

The risk in the intervention group (and its 95% confidence interval) is based on the assumed risk in the comparison group and the relative effect of the intervention (and its 95% CI).

Abbreviations: AE, adverse event; CHM, Chinese herbal medicine; CI, confidence interval; FEV$_1$, forced expiratory volume-one second; LCQ, Leicester cough questionnaire; MD, mean difference; PEF, peak expiratory flow; RR, risk ratio.

Notes

[a]Lower scores indicate less symptoms.

[1]Unclear sequence generation and allocation concealment; lack of blinding of participants and personnel.

[2]Small sample size.

Study references

Cough symptom score: H162, H166

Effective rate: H30, H47, H60

Adverse events: H30, H47, H60, H166

Table 5.29. Su huang zhi ke fang 苏黄止咳方 plus Inhaled Corticosteroids and Bronchodilators versus Inhaled Corticosteroids and Bronchodilators Alone

Outcome	Absolute Effect		Relative Effect (95% CI) No. of Participants and Studies	Certainty of the Evidence (GRADE)
	With CHM	**Without CHM**		
LCQ – not reported				
Cough symptom score Scale from: 0 to 12[a] Treatment duration: Mean four weeks	**0.85** Average difference: 0.75 points lower (95% CI: 0.89 to 0.62 fewer points)	**1.60**	**MD –0.75** (–0.89, –0.62) Based on data from 124 patients in two studies	⊕⊕◯◯ LOW[1,2]
FEV$_1$ – not reported				
PEF – not reported				
Effective rate Treatment duration: Range two to eight weeks	**76** per 100 Difference: 14 more per 100 patients (95% CI: 1 fewer to 33 more per 100 patients)	**62** per 100	**RR 1.23** (0.98 to 1.53) Based on data from 459 patients in five studies	⊕⊕◯◯ LOW[1,3]
Adverse events Based on data from 558 patients in six studies	Integrative CHM group had a total of two AEs, including gastrointestinal discomfort (one case) and dizziness (one case). The ICS plus bronchodilator groups reported eight AEs; the most common were dizziness (three cases) and chest tightness (three cases).			

The risk in the intervention group (and its 95% confidence interval) is based on the assumed risk in the comparison group and the relative effect of the intervention (and its 95% CI).

Abbreviations: AE, adverse event; CHM, Chinese herbal medicine; CI, confidence interval; FEV$_1$, forced expiratory volume-one second; ICS, inhaled corticosteroids; LCQ, Leicester cough questionnaire; MD, mean difference; PEF, peak expiratory flow; RR, risk ratio.

Notes
[a]Lower scores indicate less symptoms.
[1]Unclear sequence generation and allocation concealment; lack of blinding of participants and personnel.
[2]Small sample size.
[3]Considerable statistical heterogeneity.

Study references
Cough symptom score: H162, H166
Effective rate: H74, H100, H134, H155, H156
Adverse events: H84, H100, H134, H155, H156, H166

Zhi Sou San 止嗽散

Zhi sou san 止嗽散 was evaluated in nine studies (H52, H73, H83, H103, H106, H119, H136, H150, H157). *Zhi sou san* improved FEV_1 and was superior to pharmacotherapy in three studies with 418 participants (MD: 0.36 L [0.25, 0.47]; I^2 = 0.0%). In terms of PEF L/S, three studies (*n* = 418) combined *Zhi sou san* with pharmacotherapy and this was superior to pharmacotherapy alone (MD: 0.84 L/S [0.45, 1.23]; I^2 = 54.0%). *Zhi sou san* plus pharmacotherapy decreased EOS but there was no difference compared to pharmacotherapy alone in one study with 120 participants (MD: –0.00 ×10^9/L [–0.06, 0.05]). Total effective rate was better in the *Zhi sou san* group when it was given alone or combined with pharmacotherapy (RR: 1.31 [1.04, 1.66]; I^2 = 47.9%) and (RR 1.22 [1.11, 1.33]; I^2 = 5.3%) respectively.

Adverse events

Four studies reported adverse events. Events in the treatment group included numb lips or itching (two cases) and oropharyngeal stimulation (one case). The control group had a total of 72 adverse events including hoarseness (two cases), numb lips or itching (one case), and oropharyngeal stimulation (one case).

Xiao Qing Long Tang 小青龙汤

Xiao qing long tang 小青龙汤 was evaluated in six studies (H12, H13, H71, H90, H99, H123). It was superior to pharmacotherapy in terms of reducing the cough symptom score in one study with 59 participants (MD: –0.55 points [–0.85, –0.24]) and FEV_1 L in another study with 80 participants (MD: 1.07 L [0.88, 1.25]). *Xiao qing long tang* improved total effective rate more than pharmacotherapy alone in three studies with 164 participants (RR: 1.37 [1.05, 1.80]; I^2 = 33.3%). Combined with pharmacotherapy, it was not superior to pharmacotherapy alone in three studies with 153 participants (RR: 1.04 [0.94, 1.16]; I^2 = 0.0%).

Adverse events

None of the studies reported details of any adverse events.

Wen Dan Tang 温胆汤

Wen dan tang 温胆汤 was assessed in four studies (H102, H112, H126, H127). It was superior to pharmacotherapy in terms of LCQ in three studies (n = 122), although heterogeneity was 'high' (MD: 1.86 [0.31, 3.98]; I^2 = 71.6%). It was not superior to pharmacotherapy in three studies (n = 182) that assessed total effective rate (RR: 1.29 [0.92, 1.80]; I^2 = 78.8%).

Adverse events

One study indicated that there were no adverse events in the study.

Yu Ping Feng San 玉屏风散

Yu ping feng san 玉屏风散 was evaluated in two studies. In terms of improving total effective rate, *Yu ping feng san* combined with ICS plus bronchodilator was superior to ICS plus bronchodilator alone (RR: 1.17 [1.05, 1.32]; I^2 = 0.0%).

Adverse events

Two studies compared *Yu ping feng san* plus pharmacotherapy with pharmacotherapy alone. The integrative medicine group reported 11 adverse events including vomiting (four cases), dry mouth (two cases), dental ulcer (two cases), pharyngeal discomfort (two cases) and nausea (one case). Participants in the control group had a total of nine adverse events including dental ulcer (four cases), nausea (three cases) and dry mouth (two cases).

Qu feng xuan fei fang 祛风宣肺方

Qu feng xuan fei fang 祛风宣肺方 was evaluated in two studies. In terms of improving total effective rate, *Qu feng xuan fei fang* was better than pharmacotherapy (RR: 2.09 [1.31, 3.34]; I^2 = 27.7%).

Adverse events

One study indicated that there were no adverse events.

San Ao Tang 三拗汤

San ao tang 三拗汤 plus pharmacotherapy was superior to pharmacotherapy alone in terms of total effective rate in two studies (RR: 1.22 [1.08, 1.37]; $I^2 = 0.0\%$).

Adverse events

One study reported there were no adverse events in the treatment group, but the control group reported five events including nausea and vomiting (two cases), mild headache (one case), dizziness (one case) and dry pharynx (one case).

Zhi Ke Jiao Nang 止咳胶囊

Zhi ke jiao nang 止咳胶囊 was evaluated in two studies. Combined with ICS plus theophylline, it was superior to ICS plus theophylline alone in terms of total effective rate (RR: 1.64 [1.21, 2.22]; $I^2 = 0.0\%$).

Adverse events

None of the studies reported details of any adverse events.

Frequently Reported Herbs in Meta-analyses Showing Favourable Effect

The most frequently used herbs in meta-analyses showing favourable effect were calculated according to outcome category and comparator type. Table 5.30 includes the list of herbs.

Table 5.30. Frequently Reported Herbs in Meta-Analyses Showing Favourable Effect

Outcome Category	No. of Meta-Analyses (Studies)	Herbs	Scientific Name	Frequency of Use
Cough symptom scores*	6 (39)	*Gan cao* 甘草 inc. *zhi gan cao* 炙甘草	*Glycyrrhiza* spp.	23
		Chan tui 蝉蜕	*Cryptotympana pustulata* Fabricius	20
		Jie geng 桔梗	*Platycodon grandiflorum* (Jacq.) A. DC.	18
		Ma huang 麻黄	*Ephedra sinica* Stapf	18
		Xing ren 杏仁	*Prunus armeniaca* L. var. *ansu* Maxim.	18
		Di long 地龙	*Pheretima* spp.	15
		Chen pi 陈皮	*Citrus reticulata* Blanco	13
		Qian hu 前胡	*Peucedanum praeruptorum* Dunn	11
		Zi su zi 紫苏子	*Perilla frutescens* (L.) Britt. (fruit)	11
		Fang feng 防风	*Saposhnikovia divaricata* (Turcz.) Schischk.	10
		Zi su ye 紫苏叶	*Perilla frutescens* (L.) Britt. (leaf)	10
		Wu wei zi 五味子	*Schisandra chinensis* (Turcz.) Baill.	10
Effective rate†	2 (151)	*Gan cao* 甘草 inc. *zhi gan cao* 炙甘草	*Glycyrrhiza* spp.	98
		Ma huang 麻黄	*Ephedra sinica* Stapf	77
		Chan tui 蝉蜕	*Cryptotympana pustulata* Fabricius	70

(*Continued*)

Table 5.30. (*Continued*)

Outcome Category	No. of Meta-Analyses (Studies)	Herbs	Scientific Name	Frequency of Use
		Xing ren 杏仁	*Prunus armeniaca* L. var. *ansu* Maxim.	70
		Di long 地龙	*Pheretima* spp.	61
		Jie geng 桔梗	*Platycodon grandiflorum* (Jacq.) A. DC.	58
		Wu wei zi 五味子	*Schisandra chinensis* (Turcz.) Baill.	50
		Zi wan 紫菀	*Aster tataricus* L. f.	43
		Bai bu 百部	*Stemona* spp.	40
		Zi su ye 紫苏叶	*Perilla frutescens* (L.) Britt. (leaf)	39
Lung function‡	4 (51)	*Gan cao* 甘草 inc. *zhi gan cao* 炙甘草	*Glycyrrhiza* spp.	29
		Chan tui 蝉蜕	*Cryptotympana pustulata* Fabricius	25
		Di long 地龙	*Pheretima* spp.	24
		Jie geng 桔梗	*Platycodon grandiflorum* (Jacq.) A. DC.	24
		Ma huang 麻黄	*Ephedra sinica* Stapf	24
		Xing ren 杏仁	*Prunus armeniaca* L. var. *ansu* Maxim.	21
		Wu wei zi 五味子	*Schisandra chinensis* (Turcz.) Baill.	19
		Ban xia 半夏	*Pinellia ternata* (Thunb.) Breit.	13
		Chen pi 陈皮	*Citrus reticulata* Blanco	13
		Qian hu 前胡	*Peucedanum praeruptorum* Dunn	13

*Cough symptom scores including cough symptom score, Leicester cough questionnaire and visual analogue scales: Refer to Tables 5.4, 5.5, 5.6, 5.7, 5.8.

†Effective rate: Refer to Tables 5.22 and 5.23.

‡Lung function includes forced expiratory volume in one second (FEV_1), forced vial capacity (FVC) and peak expiratory flow (PEF): Refer to Tables 5.9, 5.10, 5.13, 5.16, 5.17.

The use of some herbs may be restricted in some countries. Readers are advised to comply with relevant regulations.

Safety of Chinese Herbal Medicine in Randomised Controlled Trials

Out of the 166 studies, 59 studies (H2, H3, H6–8, H14, H16, H19, H28, H30, H33, H37, H40, H41, H47, H53, H56, H58, H60, H61, H64, H65, H67, H68, H81, H82, H84, H85, H88, H89, H91, H92, H96–98, H100, H102, H104, H105, H113, H116, H119, H122, H129, H132–134, H138, H144, H148, H149, H151, H154–156, H158, H160, H161, H166) mentioned adverse events. Of these, 26 studies (H7, H14, H16, H28, H33, H41, H53, H61, H68, H82, H85, H89, H91, H92, H100, H102, H105, H122, H129, H132, H138, H148, H151, H155, H156, H160) reported no adverse events occurring in treatment or control groups. The remaining 33 studies (H2, H3, H6, H8, H19, H30, H37, H40, H47, H56, H58, H60, H64, H65, H67, H81, H84, H88, H96–98, H104, H113, H116, H119, H133, H134, H144, H149, H154, H158, H161, H166) provided specific details about the adverse events; one (H161) did not clarify the specific adverse events.

Chinese Herbal Medicine versus Pharmacotherapy

In 25 studies (H7, H8, H19, H30, H40, H47, H53, H60, H68, H81, H88, H89, H98, H102, H104, H113, H129, H132, H133, H138, H144, H148, H160, H161, H166) comparing CHM with pharmacotherapy, 23 adverse events were reported in people who received CHM (H30, H40, H98, H104, H113, H133, H144, H166), and 45 adverse events were reported in people taking the control pharmacotherapies (H8, H19, H40, H47, H60, H81, H88, H98, H104, H133, H144, H166). Events included hoarseness, nausea, dizziness, dry mouth, palpitation, diarrhoea and abnormal liver function test results. Eleven studies (H7, H53, H68, H89, H102, H129, H132, H138, H148, H160, H161) reported no adverse events in the treatment or control groups. Hoarseness and nausea were the most common adverse events (eight cases), followed by abdominal distension (seven cases), palpitation (seven cases), dizziness (seven cases), abnormal liver function (six cases) and diarrhoea (six cases).

Chinese Herbal Medicine plus Pharmacotherapy versus Pharmacotherapy

A total of 37 studies (H2, H3, H6, H14, H16, H28, H33, H37, H41, H56, H58, H61, H64, H65, H67, H82, H84, H85, H91, H92, H96, H97, H100, H105, H116, H119, H122, H134, H149, H151, H154, H155, H156, H158, H160, H161, H166) assessed adverse events. Fifty adverse events were reported in people who received CHM plus pharmacotherapy (H2, H3, H56, H58, H64, H65, H67, H84, H96, H97, H116, H119, H134, H149, H154, H158) and 115 adverse events were reported in people who received pharmacotherapy alone (H2, H3, H6, H37, H56, H58, H64, H65, H67, H96, H97, H116, H119, H134, H149, H154, H158, H161). Events included sleepiness, nausea, dental ulcer, dizziness, palpitations, dry mouth and abnormal renal function. Eighteen studies (H14, H16, H28, H33, H41, H61, H82, H85, H91, H92, H100, H105, H122, H151, H155, H156, H160, H166) reported that adverse events did not occur in either group. Sleepiness and nausea were the most commonly reported adverse events (19 cases), followed by dizziness (18 cases), dental ulcers (15 cases), dry mouth (ten cases), palpitation (six cases) and diarrhoea (six cases).

Controlled Clinical Trials of Chinese Herbal Medicine for Cough Variant Asthma

Controlled clinical trials are similar to an RCT but the participants are not randomly assigned to a treatment or control group. Two CCTs (H169, H170) investigated the effect of CHM versus pharmacotherapy for CVA in 163 participants. Two studies (H171, H172) evaluated CHM plus montelukast versus montelukast alone in 198 participants, one study (H167) evaluated CHM combined with ICS plus bronchodilator versus ICS plus bronchodilator alone in 85 participants, and one study (H168) evaluated CHM plus theophylline versus theophylline alone in 88 participants.

Treatment duration ranged from two to eight weeks. Five different formulas were used in the studies (Table 5.31). All

Table 5.31.   Formulas in Controlled Clinical Trials

Most Common Formulas	No. of Studies	Ingredients
Su feng tong luo fang 疏风通络方	1	*Zhi pi pa ye* 炙枇杷叶, *su ye* 苏叶, *di long* 地龙, *fang feng* 防风, *chan tui* 蝉蜕, *niu bang zi* 牛蒡子, *jing jie* 荆芥 and *gui zhi* 桂枝 (H168)
Shu feng zhi ke san 疏风止咳散	1	*Bai qian* 白前, *jie geng* 桔梗, *zi wan* 紫菀, *bai bu* 百部, *chen pi* 陈皮, *xing ren* 杏仁, *su ye* 苏叶, *chan tui* 蝉蜕 and *gan cao* 甘草 (H169)
Modified *zhi sou san* 止嗽散加减	1	*Zhi ma huang* 炙麻黄, *xing ren* 杏仁, *jie geng* 桔梗, *qian hu* 前胡, *zhi ke* 枳壳, *zi su zi* 紫苏子, *zhi pi pa ye* 炙枇杷叶, *di long* 地龙, zi wan 紫菀, chan tui 蝉蜕, wu wei zi 五味子, bai qian 白前, sha shen 沙参, bai bu 百部 and *zhi gan cao* 炙甘草 (H170)
Su huang zhi ke jiao nang 苏黄止咳胶囊	1	*Ma huang* 麻黄, *su ye* 苏叶, *di long* 地龙, *zhi pi pa ye* 炙枇杷叶, *zi su zi* 紫苏子, *chan tui* 蝉蜕, *qian hu* 前胡, *niu bang zi* 牛蒡子 and *wu wei zi* 五味子 (H171)
Feng ke fang 风咳方	1	Sang bai pi 桑白皮, xing ren 杏仁, huang qin 黄芩, *zi wan* 紫菀, *kuan dong hua* 款冬花, *qian hu* 前胡, *niu bang zi* 牛蒡子, *chan tui* 蝉蜕, *jie geng* 桔梗, *wu wei zi* 五味子 and *gan cao* 甘草 (H172)

formulas were orally administrated. Twenty-four herbs were used in the formulas and the most common was *chan tui* 蝉蜕 (Table 5.32). The controls included montelukast in three studies (H169, H171, H172), budesonide and formoterol in one study (H167), salbutamol in one study (H170) and theophylline in one study (H168).

Cough Symptom Score

One study (H172), with 100 participants, evaluated cough symptom score. The CHM plus montelukast was better than montelukast

Table 5.32. Frequently Reported Herbs in Controlled Clinical Trials

Most Common Herbs	Scientific Name	Frequency of Use
Chan tui 蝉蜕	*Cryptotympana pustulata Fabricius.*	5
Zhi pi pa ye 炙枇杷叶	*Folia eriobotryae.*	3
Niu bang zi 牛蒡子	*Arctium lappa* L.	3
Jie geng 桔梗	*Platycodon grandiflorum (Jacq.) A. DC.*	3
Zi wan 紫菀	*Aster tataricus L. f.*	3
Xing ren 杏仁	*Prunus armeniaca* L. var. *ansu* Maxim.	3
Wu wei zi 五味子	*Schisandra chinensis (Turcz.) Baill.*	3
Qian hu 前胡	*Peucedanum praeruptorum* Dunn.	3
Di long 地龙	*Pheretima spp.*	3
Su ye 苏叶	*Perilla frutescens* (L.) Britt. (leaf).	3
Gan cao/zhi gan cao 甘草 (炙)	*Glycyrrhiza spp.*	3

alone and decreased cough symptom score (MD: −0.18 points [−0.27, −0.09]).

Forced Expiratory Volume in One Second

One study (H167), with 85 participants, assessed FEV_1 L. The CHM combined with ICS plus bronchodilator was more effective than ICS plus bronchodilator alone (MD: 0.18 L [0.04, 0.31]). One study (H172), with 100 participants, assessed FEV_1 %. The CHM combined with montelukast was not superior to montelukast alone (MD: −1.99% [−4.93, 0.95]).

Peak Expiratory Flow

Two studies measured lung function using PEF. One study (H170), with 91 participants, assessed the effect of CHM compared with Ventolin® and found that CHM was superior to Ventolin® (MD: 4.05 % [0.15, 7.94]). One study (H172), with 100 participants, evaluated the effect of CHM plus montelukast, and it was found to be not superior to montelukast alone (MD: −0.97 % [−3.71, 1.77]).

Total Effective Rate

Five studies measured the total effective rate. Two studies (H169, H170) (*n* = 163) evaluated the effect of CHM compared with pharmacotherapy, and CHM was superior to pharmacotherapy (RR: 1.29 [1.07, 1.54]; I^2 = 0.0%). Three studies (H167, H168, H171) (*n* = 271) assessed the effect of CHM plus pharmacotherapy, compared with pharmacotherapy alone, and CHM plus pharmacotherapy was better, although heterogeneity was 'high' (RR: 1.40 [1.02, 1.94]; I^2 = 72.5%).

Safety of Chinese Herbal Medicine in Controlled Clinical Trials

One of the six studies, with 98 participants (H171), assessed the safety of CHM plus montelukast for CVA. Rash (three cases), nausea (one case) and constipation (one case) were reported in participants using CHM plus montelukast, while 11 adverse events were reported in the montelukast group including nausea (five cases), constipation (four cases), and rash (two cases).

Non-controlled Studies of Chinese Herbal Medicine for Cough Variant Asthma

Eight non-controlled studies (H173–H180) evaluated CHM in 656 participants with CVA. Treatment duration ranged from ten days to six weeks. All studies assessed oral CHM alone, including one study (H176) using Chinese patent medicines such as *Xiao qing long granule* 小青龙颗粒剂. Seven assessed herbal decoctions including *Zhi sou san* 止嗽散 （H178）, *She gan ma huang tang* 射干麻黄汤 (H173), *Xuan fei zhi sou tang* 宣肺止嗽汤 (H174), *Feng ke tang* 风咳汤 (H175), *Xiao qing long tang* 小青龙汤 (H177), *Xuan fei ping chuan fang* 宣肺平喘方 (H179) and *Xuan fei hua tan zhi ke fang* 宣肺化痰平喘止咳方 (H180). *Xiao qing long tang* 小青龙汤 was the only formula used in more than one study (H176, H177). Forty-one herbs were used in the formulas, and the most common were *ma huang* 麻黄, *xing ren* 杏仁, *gan cao* 甘草, *zi wan* 紫菀, *chan tui* 蝉蜕

and *wu wei zi* 五味子. None of the studies reported details of any adverse events.

Clinical Evidence for Commonly Used Chinese Herbal Medicine Treatments

The CHMs recommended in clinical practice guidelines (see Chapter 2 for the complete list) have been evaluated in RCTs. The formula *Su huang zhi ke fang* 苏黄止咳方 was used in 25 studies (H15, H29, H30, H43, H47, H49, H55, H60, H74, H84, H89, H96, H97, H100, H116, H134, H138, H143, H154–H156, H159, H162, H166, H171) and the results are reported in the previous section. Another formula, *Xu fu dai zhe tang* 旋覆代赭汤, has been evaluated in one study (H39). The results showed that *Xu fu dai zhe tang* 旋覆代赭汤 was superior to bronchodilators in terms of total effective rate (RR: 2.3 [1.31, 4.01]) and reduced EOS (MD: -0.06×10^9/L [-0.13, 0.01]). Other formulas recommended in guidelines were not found in this analysis.

Chinese Herbal Medicine for Upper Airways Cough Syndrome

Chinese herbal medicine for UACS was researched in 14 studies. The results of these studies are analysed and discussed in separate sections below for the 11 RCTs (H181–H191), one CCT (H192) and two non-controlled studies (H193, H194).

Randomised Controlled Trials of Chinese Herbal Medicine for Upper Airways Cough Syndrome

The UACS studies were conducted in China between 2010 and 2017. The studies included 1,201 participants and treatment duration ranged from ten days to four weeks. Chinese medicine syndrome classification was used in six studies. The reported syndromes were as follows:

- Severe wind attacking the Lungs 风盛挛急 (two studies);
- Wind-heat attacking the Lungs 风热犯肺 (two studies);

- Wind-cold attacking the Lungs 风寒袭肺 (one study);
- Wind-phlegm obstructing the Lungs 风痰阻肺 (one study).

Herbal formulas were self-designed in all studies, except three that used *Zhi sou san* 止嗽散, *Ma huang xi xin fu zi tang* 麻黄细辛附子汤 or *Ke ping tang* 咳平汤. All formulas were administered orally with decoction or granule powder. A total of 53 distinct herbs were used in the formulas and the most common (used in five or more studies) were *jie geng* 桔梗 (nine studies), *ma huang* 麻黄 (eight studies), *gan cao* 甘草 (six studies), *xing ren* 杏仁 (six studies), *bai qian* 白前 (five studies) and *jing jie* 荆芥 (five studies).

Risk of Bias

All studies specified that 'randomisation' was used in the allocation of participants to the CHM intervention or the control groups. However, only two studies clearly specified the method of random sequence generation and none of the studies described the method of allocation concealment and were thus judged to be at 'unclear' risk of bias. Two studies used a placebo control and blinded participants and personnel. Other studies lacked information about blinding of participants and personnel and were at 'high' risk of bias. Incomplete outcome data was assessed at 'low' risk of bias because there was no missing data and drop-outs were balanced between groups. Study protocols were not identified for any of the studies (either in electronic databases or clinical trial registries); therefore, studies were judged to be at 'unclear' risk of bias for selective reporting. The risk of bias is summarised in Table 5.33.

Outcomes

Outcomes included the LCQ,[10] cough symptom score,[11–13] and total effective rate.[16–17] The most common outcome was total effective rate used in all studies. Other outcomes, such as FEV_1, PEF, FeNO, blood eosinophil count, eosinophil cationic protein and cough reflex sensitivity were not used because they are more appropriate measurements for CVA, not UACS.

Table 5.33. Risk of Bias of Randomised Controlled Trials: Upper Airways Cough Syndrome

Risk of Bias Domain	Low Risk n (%)	Unclear Risk n (%)	High Risk n (%)
Sequence generation	2 (18.2)	9 (81.8)	0 (0)
Allocation concealment	0 (0)	11 (100)	0 (0)
Blinding of participants	2 (18.2)	0 (0)	9 (81.8)
Blinding of personnel	2 (18.2)	0 (0)	9 (81.8)
Blinding of outcome assessors	0 (0)	0 (0)	11 (100)
Incomplete outcome data	11 (100)	0 (0)	0 (0)
Selective outcome reporting	0 (0)	11 (100)	0 (0)

In the following sections the meta-analysis results are presented according to the outcome measure. For each outcome, studies are grouped by comparator, for instance, CHM versus placebo, CHM versus pharmacotherapies, CHM plus pharmacotherapies versus pharmacotherapies alone as integrative medicine. Subgroup analysis was not performed because of the small number of included studies.

Leicester Cough Questionnaire

The CHM was superior to placebo in terms of LCQ scores (higher scores indicate less severe symptoms) in one study of 291 participants (MD: 0.56 [0.34, 0.78]). In addition, CHM was also superior to antihistamines and antitussives in one study of 86 participants (MD: 0.43 points [0.05, 0.81]).

Cough Symptom Score

One study ($n = 48$) assessed cough symptom score. The CHM was superior to antihistamines (lower scores indicate less symptoms) (MD: –0.84 points [–1.22, –0.46]).

Total Effective Rate

When CHM was compared to placebo, total effective rate was better in the CHM group (RR: 1.77 [1.32, 2.37], $I^2 = 0.00\%$, two studies,

n = 331). Seven studies (n = 738) evaluated CHM compared to pharmacotherapies and total effective rate; there was no difference between groups (RR: 1.17 [0.98, 1.39]). When CHM was combined with pharmacotherapies and compared to pharmacotherapies alone, there was no difference between groups (RR: 1.39 [0.75, 2.57], I^2 = 74%).

Controlled Clinical Trials of Chinese Herbal Medicine for Upper Airways Cough Syndrome

One CCT (H192) assessed CHM for UACS. A total of 109 participants had the CM syndrome *Shao Yang* syndrome 邪客少阳证 and were given modified *Xiao chai hu tang* 小柴胡汤 （加减）plus an antihistamine, antitussive and expectorant, compared to the antihistamine, antitussive and expectorant alone for two weeks. Total effective rate was measured and showed that the integrative medicine was not superior to the control (RR: 1.21 [0.95, 1.55]). The study did not report adverse event data.

Non-controlled Studies of Chinese Herbal Medicine for Upper Airways Cough Syndrome

Two non-controlled studies assessed CHM; one assessed *Shu feng li yan zhi ke tang* 疏风利咽止咳汤 for two to four weeks and the other assessed *Wen fei zhi liu dan* 温肺止流丹 for 10–30 days. Neither of the studies reported details of any adverse events.

Chinese Herbal Medicine for Gastro-oesophageal Reflux Disease-related Cough

Chinese herbal medicine for GORD-C was assessed in 18 studies. The results of these studies are analysed and discussed in separate sections below for 16 RCTs (H195–H210), and two non-controlled studies (H211, H212).

Randomised Controlled Trials of Chinese Herbal Medicine for Gastro-oesophageal Reflux Disease-related Cough

All studies were conducted in China between 2008 and 2017. The studies included 1,247 participants and treatment duration ranged from 15 days to 12 weeks. Chinese medicine syndrome classification was used in two studies and included Liver depression, Spleen deficiency 肝郁脾虚 and Stomach *qi* ascending 胃气上逆.

All formulas were orally administered decoctions. Five studies administered a self-designed formula, and the other 11 studies administered different herbal formulas including the following:

- *Si ni san* 四逆散 (three studies);
- *Ban xia hou po tang* 半夏厚朴汤 (two studies);
- *An wei zhi ke jian* 安胃止咳煎 (one study);
- *Zhi sou san* and *ban xia xie xin tang* 止嗽散合半夏泻心汤 (one study);
- *Sang ju qing jie tang* 桑菊清解汤 (one study);
- *Chai hu shu gan san* 柴胡疏肝散 (one study);
- *Wen wei jiang ni ke li* 温胃降逆颗粒 (one study);
- *He wei wen dan tang* 和胃温胆汤 (one study).

A total of 66 distinct herbs were used in the formulas. Most herbs were used in one or two studies and only five herbs were used in five or more studies, including *chai hu* 柴胡 (nine studies), *gan cao* 甘草 (nine studies), *ban xia* 半夏 (eight studies), *bai shao* 白芍 (seven studies) and *fu ling* 茯苓 (six studies).

Risk of Bias

All studies specified that 'randomisation' was used in the allocation of participants to the CHM intervention or the control groups. However, only six studies clearly specified the method of random sequence generation and one used concealed envelopes as the method of allocation concealment; none of the other studies described the method of allocation concealment and were judged

Table 5.34. Risk of Bias of Randomised Controlled Trials: Gastro-oesophageal Reflux Disease-related Cough

Risk of Bias Domain	Low Risk *n* (%)	Unclear Risk *n* (%)	High Risk *n* (%)
Sequence generation	6 (37.5)	10 (62.5)	0 (0)
Allocation concealment	1 (6.3)	15 (93.8)	0 (0)
Blinding of participants	0 (0)	0 (0)	16 (100)
Blinding of personnel	0 (0)	0 (0)	16 (100)
Blinding of outcome assessors	0 (0)	0 (0)	16 (100)
Incomplete outcome data	16 (100)	0 (0)	0 (0)
Selective outcome reporting	0 (0)	15 (93.8)	1 (6.3)

to be at 'unclear' risk of bias. Studies lacked information about blinding of participants and personnel and were at 'high' risk of bias. Incomplete outcome data was assessed at 'low' risk of bias because there was no missing data and drop-outs were balanced between groups. Study protocols were not identified for any of the studies (either in electronic databases or clinical trial registries); therefore, studies were judged to be at 'unclear' risk of bias for selective reporting, except one study that did not report results from one outcome and was judged to be at 'high' risk of bias. The risk of bias is summarised in Table 5.34.

Outcomes

Outcomes for GORD-C included those typically seen with other chronic cough clinical trials such as the LCQ,[10] cough symptom score[11–13] and total effective rate.[16,17] Lung function, exhaled nitric oxide and eosinophil counts were not measured because the pathophysiology of GORD-C differs from CVA and UACS, and these outcomes are not good indicators of disease progression or treatment effect.

Alongside the cough questionnaires, the reflux disease questionnaire was used in some GORD-C studies. It is a 12-item self-administered questionnaire, that measures the GORD component, rather than cough, in terms of frequency and severity of heartburn, regurgitation and dyspeptic complaints.[18] In the following sections the meta-analysis results are presented according to the outcome measure. For each outcome, studies are grouped by comparator, for instance, CHM versus pharmacotherapies and CHM plus pharmacotherapies versus pharmacotherapies as integrative medicine. Subgroup analysis was not performed because of the small number of included studies.

Leicester Cough Questionnaire

The CHM alone or combined with pharmacotherapies was assessed in five studies (H198, H201, H203, H207, H208). Pharmacotherapies included proton pump inhibitors (PPI) and drugs to promote gastrointestinal motility, such as mosapride, domperidone and lansoprazole. The CHM was superior to pharmacotherapies in four studies (318 participants) (MD: 1.90 [0.82, 2.98], $I^2 = 71\%$). The CHM plus a PPI and domperidone (promotes gastric motility) versus PPI and domperidone alone showed a significant improvement favouring the CHM group in one study with 82 participants (MD: 2.10 [1.97, 2.23]).

Cough Symptom Score

Five studies, including 446 participants, assessed cough symptom score (H198, H199, H201, H203, H206). The CHM was superior to pharmacotherapies (SMD: –0.91 [–1.22, –0.46], $I^2 = 80\%$). One study compared CHM plus a PPI and domperidone to the PPI and domperidone alone; the CHM group was superior to control and reduced the cough symptom score (MD: –0.80 [–1.21, –0.39]).

Visual Analogue Scales

One study, including 64 participants, used a VAS to assess symptoms (H200) at the end of treatment based on different comparators. The

CHM plus a PPI and mosapride (accelerates gastric emptying), compared to PPI and mosapride alone, reduced symptoms on the VAS scale (MD: –1.98 [–2.90, –1.06]).

Reflux Disease Questionnaire

One study, including 64 participants, reported results from the reflux disease questionnaire (H200). There were no differences in results between CHM plus pharmacotherapy versus pharmacotherapy alone in one study (MD: –0.12 [–1.40, 1.16]).

Total Effective Rate

All 16 RCTs assessed effective rate. In 13 studies that compared CHM to pharmacotherapies, results showed that CHM improved symptoms more than control (RR: 1.42 [1.19, 1.70], $I^2 = 76\%$). Integrative medicine, including CHM and pharmacotherapy, was superior to pharmacotherapy alone in three studies (RR: 1.66 [1.32, 2.10], $I^2 = 0\%$).

Non-controlled Studies of Chinese Herbal Medicine for Gastro-oesophageal Reflux Disease-related Cough

Two non-controlled studies (H211, H212) including 86 participants assessed CHM. One assessed the CHM formulas *Er chen tang* 二陈汤 and *Zhi sou san* 止嗽散 plus a PPI and antibiotic for four weeks. The other study used *He wei zhi sou tang* 和胃止嗽汤 without any pharmacotherapies for 10–30 days. The studies did not report details of adverse events.

Summary of Chinese Herbal Medicine Clinical Evidence

Over 200 studies have assessed the benefits and safety of CHM alone, or combined with pharmacotherapies, for CVA, UACS and

GORD-C. Cough variant asthma is the most commonly assessed subtype in the included literature, accounting for 83.4%. This is not surprising as CVA is a common condition in China; most of the included literature is published in Mandarin and includes Chinese participants. Upper airway cough syndrome was less common due to variability in diagnosis across different regions as well as recent changes in terminology, such as the removal of postnasal drip syndrome in international clinical guidelines. Similarly, GORD-C is difficult to diagnose, and only more recently has it become a frequently cited cause of chronic cough.

Chinese medicine syndromes were reported in CVA and UACS studies and often included wind alongside other pathogens such as heat, phlegm and cold. Deficiency syndromes included *qi* and *yin*. Gastro-oesophageal reflux disease-related cough syndromes were different and included Stomach and Liver patterns. The CHM formulas and herbal ingredients were similar among all subtypes of chronic cough. For example, *Zhi sou san* 止嗽散 formula and the herbs *chen pi* 陈皮, *gan cao* 甘草 and *xing ren* 杏仁 were in the top 20 lists of CVA, UACS and GORD-C. Differences were also observed, for example CVA and UACS studies more commonly used *ma huang* 麻黄, *jing jie* 荆芥, *jie geng* 桔梗 and *fang feng* 防风, compared to GORD-C studies that used *chai hu* 柴胡, *bai zhu* 白术, *bai shao* 白芍 and *fu ling* 茯苓. Most of the studies assessed the effects of CHM over the short term and only 29 RCTs (14.6%) had a duration of six weeks or more, which limits the ability to generalise the results because CVA, UACS and GORD-C often require long-term treatment.

Pharmacotherapies were used as control in most of the studies (placebo used in three studies) and CHM was given alongside pharmacotherapies in about half of the studies. The pharmacotherapies were consistent with those recommended in conventional medicine clinical practice guidelines. Pharmacotherapies differed among the subtypes of chronic cough, which is not surprising as the treatments for these conditions vary. Pharmacotherapies for CVA often included ICS, bronchodilators and leukotriene receptor antagonists (montelukast). Antihistamines and theophylline were less commonly used and are not generally recommended as first-line therapy for CVA. The pharmacotherapies for UACS were slightly different and seldom included ICS and bronchodilators, but almost always included antihistamines and antitussives (montelukast). The profile of GORD-C pharmacotherapies and control interventions were different again and included PPI in all studies and drugs that promote gastrointestinal motility in most studies.

Chinese herbal medicine alone or combined with pharmacotherapies improved symptoms of cough in terms of reducing scores on the LCQ, the cough symptom score, 10-point VAS and total effective rate in all subtypes of chronic cough. In terms of outcomes specific for CVA, CHM improved lung function and cough reflex sensitivity as well as PEF when CHM was combined with pharmacotherapies. The CHM alone or given as integrative medicine did not significantly change eosinophil counts. Results from the CVA studies were analysed using the GRADE approach and the certainty of the evidence was found to be 'low' to 'very low'.

Despite the positive results, the studies were not free from bias and heterogeneity was 'high' in most of the meta-analyses results. Therefore, all results presented in this chapter should be cautiously interpreted to not overestimate the potential beneficial effect of CHM for chronic cough. Safety outcomes, such as adverse events, were reported in about one-third of studies (32.6%). Overall, CHM appeared to be safe for people with chronic cough when taken alone or alongside other pharmacotherapies. The number of adverse events was generally less in the CHM groups and overall mild in nature and self-resolving.

References

1. 马锦地, 谢洋, 李建生. (2015) 苏黄止咳胶囊治疗咳嗽变异性哮喘的 Meta分析. 中医学 报 **30(04):** 477–480.

2. 卜松其,夏清青, 张宇锋. (2016) 苏黄止咳胶囊治疗咳嗽变异性哮喘的系统评价. 中医学报 **31(07):** 965–967.

3. 吴丽华, 蒋红丽, 闵捷, *et al.* (2015) 中药治疗咳嗽变异性哮喘的系统评价. 中国循证医学杂志. **15(09):** 1084–1089.

4. 戴磊, 黎伟林, 黎志刚. (2017) 中医药治疗咳嗽变异性哮喘随机对照试验的Meta分析. 中国医学创新 **14(08):** 21–27.

5. 陈伦, 祁佳, 张宇锋, 江卫龙. (2016) 黄芪细辛汤治疗咳嗽变异性哮喘的系统评价. 世界中医药 **11(01):** 155–158.

6. 潘宝峰,李秀娟, 张伟伟, *et al.* (2017) 桂枝加厚朴杏子汤治疗咳嗽变异型哮喘临床疗效的Meta分析. 中医药导报 **23(19):** 106–108.

7. 吴科锐, 罗景山, 李林蔓, *et al.* (2017) 加味小柴胡汤治疗咳嗽变异性哮喘的Meta分析. 中国医药指南 **15(24):** 3–4.

8. Jiang H, Liu W, Li G, *et al.* (2016) Chinese medicinal herbs in the treatment of upper airway cough syndrome: A systematic review of randomized, controlled trials. *Altern Ther Health Med* **22(3):** 38–51.

9. Zhao YH, Liu ZI, Li LH, *et al.* (2012) Systematic review of randomized controlled trials of traditional Chinese medicine treatment of non-acute bronchial asthma complicated by gastroesophageal reflux. *J Tradit Chin Med* **32(1):** 12–18.

10. Birring SS, Prudon B, Carr AJ, *et al.* (2003) Development of a symptom specific health status measure for patients with chronic cough: Leicester Cough Questionnaire (LCQ). *Thorax* **58:** 339–343.

11. Asthma Workgroup of Chinese Society of Respiratory Diseases (CSRD), Chinese Medical Association. (2011) The Chinese national guidelines on diagnosis and management of cough (December 2010). *Chin Med J* **124:** 3207–3219.

12. Hsu JY, Stone RA, Logan-Sinclair RB, *et al.* (1994) Coughing frequency in patients with persistent cough: Assessment using a 24-hour ambulatory recorder. *Eur Respir J* **7:** 1246–1253.

13. Chung KF. (2006) Measurement of cough. *Respir Physiol Neurobiol* **152:** 329–339.

14. Raed A, Peter B, Serpil C, *et al.* (2011) An Official ATS Clinical Practice Guideline: Interpretation of Exhaled nitric oxide levels (FENO) for clinical applications. *Am J Respir Crit Care Med* **184:** 602–615.

15. Dicpinigaitis PV. (2003) Short- and long-term reproducibility of capsaicin cough challenge testing. *Pulm Pharmacol Ther* **16:** 61–65.

16. 中药新药临床研究指导原则. (2013) 中华人民共和国卫生部, 人民卫生出版社.

17. 中医病症诊断疗效标准. (1995) 国家中医药管理局, 南京: 南京大学出版社.

18. Shaw MJ, Talley NJ, Beebe TJ, *et al.* (2001). Initial validation of a diagnostic questionnaire for gastroesophageal reflux disease. *Am J Gastroenterol* **96(1):** 52–57.

References for Included Chinese Herbal Medicine Clinical Studies

Study No.	Reference
H1	安巍巍, 冯胜奎. (2013) 中药治疗咳嗽变异性哮喘临床观察. 中国药物经济学 **(S3):** 58–60.
H2	蔡绪明, 张军城, 苏平, 曹利平. (2017) 曹氏清金化痰汤联合多索茶碱片治疗咳嗽变异性哮喘临床观察. 陕西中医药大学学报 **40(01):** 44–46.
H3	曾红萍. (2015) 加味柴胡疏肝散治疗咳嗽变异性哮喘 (肝郁证) 的临床疗效研究.成都中医药大学.
H4	曾庆霖. (2011) 风咳方治疗咳嗽变异性哮喘临床观察. 湖南中医药大学.
H5	曾小芹. (2017) 宣肺平喘止咳方联合孟鲁司特钠对发作期咳嗽变异性哮喘患者血清 IgE, IL-4 和 TNF-α 水平的影响. 现代中西医结合杂志 **26(14):** 1536–1538.
H6	常力. (2016) 咳喘胶囊联合舒利迭治疗咳嗽变异型哮喘 19 例. 河南中医 **36(03):** 496–498.
H7	陈凤兰, 陈粉莲, 卢杰宁, 萧汉达, 邝宁子, 李轩. (2014) 消风止嗽汤治疗咳嗽变异性哮喘随机平行对照研究. 实用中医内科杂志 **28(07):** 26–28.
H8	陈黎, 李红. (2008) 消风活血, 润肺利气法治疗咳嗽变异性哮喘. 浙江中西医结合杂志 **18(12):** 729–730, 733.
H9	陈世伟, 李卫青, 李巨奇, 王建国. (2016) 加味参附姜苓汤对围月经期咳嗽变异性哮喘患者血清 MMP-2, MMP-9 及 TIMP-1 表达的影响. 湖南中医药大学学报 **36(02):** 65–67, 75.
H10	陈艳华. (2016) 祛风止咳汤治疗咳嗽变异性哮喘临床研究. 山东中医杂志. **35(01):** 31–33.
H11	陈洋凯. (2011) 止咳胶囊治疗咳嗽变异性哮喘气阴两虚型的临床研究. 山东中医药大学.
H12	陈媛丽. (2013) 小青龙汤加味治疗寒饮伏肺型咳嗽变异性哮喘的疗效观察. 广州中医药大学.

(*Continued*)

(Continued)

Study No.	Reference
H13	陈媛丽, 李慧. (2012) 小青龙汤加味治疗咳嗽变异性哮喘疗效观察. 亚太传统医药 **8(12):** 40–41.
H14	陈月宁, 翁小光. (2016) 疏风通络方在风痰型咳嗽变异性哮喘治疗中的效果观察. 内蒙古中医药 **35(15):** 10–11.
H15	成建芬, 韩继红, 苏方芳. (2014) 苏黄止咳胶囊联合富马酸酮替芬治疗咳嗽变异性哮喘的临床观察. 白求恩医学杂志 **12(05):** 515–516.
H16	程娜娜, 侯宇辉. (2016) 半夏厚朴汤治疗咳嗽变异性哮喘的临床研究. 中医临床研究 **8(23):** 40–42.
H17	仇淑莉. (2015) 广济止咳方治疗咳嗽变异性哮喘少阳郁结证临床研究. 河南中医 **35(10):** 2454–2456.
H18	丛晓东. (2013) 温润辛金方对咳嗽变异性哮喘 (风寒恋肺型) 疗效及其生活质量的影响. 北京中医药大学.
H19	崔云. (2017) 王书臣学术思想与临床经验总结及补肾祛风法治疗咳嗽变异性哮喘临床研究. 中国中医科学院.
H20	代昭欣. (2010) 润肺止咳法治疗咳嗽变异性哮喘临床和实验研究. 中国中医科学院.
H21	戴莉娜, 陈宁. (2015) 辛麻颗粒治疗咳嗽变异性哮喘的临床观察. 按摩与康复医学 **6(10):** 95–97.
H22	刁玉明. (2016) 疏风宣肺止咳汤对CVA的疗效及对 BHR 的影响. 西南国防医药 **26(07):** 776–779.
H23	丁静, 王淑英, 杨环玮, 冯文杰. (2015) 疏风止咳方治疗咳嗽变异性哮喘 45 例临床观察. 河北中医 **37(06):** 854–856.
H24	丁念. (2010) 地龙二陈汤治疗咳嗽变异性哮喘 40 例. 陕西中医 **31(08):** 943–944.
H25	董辉. (2010) 自拟止嗽熄风散治疗咳嗽变异型哮喘临床观察. 中华实用中西医杂志 **23(5):** 1–2.
H26	范德斌, 秦雪屏, 白红华, 徐金柱, 曾艳红, 曾国强, *et al.* (2008) 中西医结合治疗咳嗽变异性哮喘102例疗效观察. 云南中医中药杂志 **29(11):** 27–28.
H27	冯德华. (2012) "祛风止痉方" 联合孟鲁司特钠治疗咳嗽变异性哮喘 40 例临床研究. 江苏中医药 **44(07):** 17–18.
H28	冯美, 张建, 王诚喜. (2014) 加味五福饮治疗咳嗽变异性哮喘 30 例临床观察. 湖南中医杂志 **30(01):** 15–17.

(*Continued*)

Study No.	Reference
H29	冯勇明, 黎颖. (2017) 苏黄止咳胶囊联合布地奈德吸入治疗咳嗽变异性哮喘效果观察. 光明中医 **32(09)**: 1331–1333.
H30	葛阳涛. (2015) 苏黄止咳胶囊治疗咳嗽变异性哮喘 (风咳) 60 例临床观察. 北京中医药大学.
H31	龚年金, 田正鉴. (2011) 中西医结合治疗咳嗽变异性哮喘临床观察. 中国中医药咨讯 **3(20)**: 471.
H32	谷春燕, 张晓雅. (2015) 润肺调中降逆汤治疗咳嗽变异性哮喘临床观察. 现代中医临床 **22(04)**: 34–37.
H33	韩秀娟. (2008) 清肝泻肺法治疗咳嗽变异性哮喘肝火犯肺型的临床研究. 山东中医药大学.
H34	韩旭东. (2012) 中西医结合治疗风邪犯肺型咳嗽变异性哮喘疗效观察. 山西中医 **28(01)**: 24–25.
H35	郝月琴, 张明泳, 郝万明. (2007) 加味玄麦甘桔汤治疗咳嗽变异性哮喘的临床观察. 中国实验方剂学杂志 **13(05)**: 57–58.
H36	侯思聪. (2017) 滋阴清热法对咳嗽变异性哮喘患者血清 IgE, IL-5 及 FeNO 的影响. 中国中医药科技 **24(04)**: 405–407, 411.
H37	胡芳, 赵立杰, 郭军英. (2016) 三拗片口服联合舒利迭吸入治疗咳嗽变异型哮喘疗效观察. 山西医药杂志 **45(04)**: 429–431.
H38	胡丽琴. (2012) 补肾益气方治疗咳嗽变异性哮喘 50 例. 中国中医药现代远程教育 **10(09)**: 14–15.
H39	胡敏, 苑惠清. (2008) 旋覆代赭汤加减治疗肺胃气逆型咳嗽变异性哮喘 32 例. 中华中西医学杂志 **6(6)**: 50–52.
H40	黄波贞, 李吉武, 王评. (2010) 加味小柴胡汤治疗咳嗽变异型哮喘临床观察. 中国中医急症 **19(09)**: 1457–1458.
H41	黄海屏. (2014) 中西医结合治疗咳嗽变异性哮喘疗效观察. 山西中医 **30(07)**: 23–24.
H42	黄青松, 肖玮, 吴建英. (2013) 敏咳煎治疗咳嗽变异性哮喘疗效观察. 新中医 **45(10)**: 23–25.
H43	黄素坤, 张国彦. (2017) 苏黄止咳胶囊联合布地奈德雾化吸入治疗咳嗽变异性哮喘的临床观察. 东南国防医药 **19(06)**: 608–610.
H44	黄召谊, 屠庆年, 陈广. (2012) 消风散联合阿斯美治疗咳嗽变异性哮喘的临床研究. 湖北中医药大学学报 **14(04)**: 44–46.

(*Continued*)

(*Continued*)

Study No.	Reference
H45	黄珍恺, 吴孝田, 赵祥安, 等. (2017) 祛风止咳汤治疗 CVA 患者 44 例临床观察. 光明中医 **32(19):** 2780–2782.
H46	吉保民, 支艳, 马建伟. (2011) 滋阴清热法对咳嗽变异性哮喘患者疗效及 ECP, IL-5 的影响. 中国中医急症 **20(02):** 199–201.
H47	贾明月. (2012) 苏黄止咳胶囊治疗咳嗽变异性哮喘的临床疗效评价. 北京中医药大学.
H48	江曙光. (2005) 疏风宣肺汤治疗咳嗽型哮喘的临床观察. 湖南中医药大学.
H49	蒋珺. (2017) 苏黄止咳胶囊联合布地奈德吸入治疗咳嗽变异性哮喘疗效观察. 现代中西医结合杂志 **26(29):** 3245–3247.
H50	金伟, 郭震兵, 董薇, 顾乃龙. (2015) 顾乃龙宣肺止嗽方治疗风邪犯肺型咳嗽变异性哮喘临床疗效观察. 新疆中医药 **33(05):** 16–18.
H51	康年松, 马伟明, 陈笑腾, 韩旭丰, 岑迎东, 劳士权, *et al.* (2017) 蝉衣合剂加减治疗咳嗽变异性哮喘临床疗效观察. 浙江中西医结合杂志 **27(02):** 123–125.
H52	李彬, 孟泳. (2015) 止嗽散和三子养亲汤联合舒利迭治疗咳嗽变异性哮喘 56 例. 中国中医药现代远程教育 **13(04):** 59–60.
H53	李才元. (2018) 自拟加味二陈汤调控咳嗽变异性哮喘患者气道神经源性炎症的作用机制研究. 现代中西医结合杂志 **27(08):** 837–840.
H54	李格, 王倩倩, 杨慧敏, 聂翠娟, 赵景曼. (2017) 麻杏祛风颗粒对咳嗽变异性哮喘患者肺功能影响. 临床医药文献电子杂志 **4(76):** 14994–14995.
H55	李金宪. (2002) 疏风宣肺法治疗咳嗽变异性哮喘的临床研究. 北京中医药大学.
H56	李康, 秦晓华. (2014) 金沸草散加减联合西药治疗咳嗽变异性哮喘 42 例. 中医杂志 **55(02):** 161–163.
H57	李丽梅, 叶焰, 刘红宇. (2017) 加味参苓白术散联合复方甲氧那明治疗脾虚湿盛型咳嗽变异性哮喘 30 例临床研究. 江苏中医药 **49(11):** 30–32.
H58	李少琳, 方燕芬, 刘巧莲, 等. (2016) 玉屏风胶囊联合舒利迭对咳嗽变异性哮喘的免疫调节作用研究. 国际中医中药杂志 **38(6):** 512–514.
H59	李松林. (2017) 自拟麻杏利咽汤治疗变异性哮喘慢性咳嗽的临床效果观察. 临床合理用药杂志 **10(32):** 37–38.
H60	李颖, 王雪京. (2013) 风咳方治疗咳嗽变异性哮喘疗效及其对血嗜酸性粒细胞和免疫球蛋白E的影响. 中国中医药信息杂志 **20(06):** 5–7.

(*Continued*)

Study No.	Reference
H61	林鸿春, 李楠, 焦扬, 等. (2016) 疏风宣肺汤治疗咳嗽变异性哮喘风邪犯肺证 42 例疗效观察. 中医临床研究 **8(15):** 12–14.
H62	刘红宇, 叶焰, 熊艳云, 李俐. (2014) 健脾肃肺方治疗咳嗽变异性哮喘临床观察. 湖北中医杂志 **36(10):** 3–4.
H63	刘宏. (2011) 补肺汤加减治疗成年人咳嗽变异性哮喘临床观察. 中国中医药信息杂志 **18(06):** 67–68.
H64	刘焰. (2016) 疏金利肺汤辅助沙美特罗/氟替卡松吸入治疗咳嗽变异性哮喘疗效观察. 现代中西医结合杂志 **25(19):** 2106–2108.
H65	柳书芬, 朱静娟, 周承朋, 等. (2016) 玉屏风颗粒辅助舒利迭治疗咳嗽变异性哮喘临床研究. 国际中医中药杂志 **38(11):** 986–988.
H66	楼静, 邬海燕, 崔恩海. (2015) 疏风止咳汤治疗咳嗽变异性哮喘临床研究. 新中医 **47(11):** 57–59.
H67	陆顺意, 黄河清. (2015) 郁热方治疗咳嗽变异性哮喘63例临床观察. 光明中医 **30(7):** 1422–1424.
H68	罗继红. (2009) 咳平汤治疗风邪犯肺型咳嗽变异性哮喘临床观察. 福建中医学院.
H69	罗社文, 张洪春, 韩春生, 李金宪, 晁恩祥. (2002) 疏风宣肺法治疗咳嗽变异性哮喘的临床观察. 中国医药学报 **17(08):** 473–475.
H70	吕献青, 谭捷, 王红艳. (2009) 桑通颗粒治疗咳嗽变异性哮喘 42 例临床观察. 河北中医 **31(02):** 184–185.
H71	马玉兰, 张海霞, 王淑芳. (2012) 小青龙汤加减治疗咳嗽变异性哮喘(风寒袭肺内有寒饮型) 40 例. 光明中医 **27(04):** 845–847.
H72	苗倩倩. (2012) 基于止嗽散合方治疗咳嗽变异性哮喘的临床研究. 北京中医药大学.
H73	苗青, 魏鹏草, 苗倩, 张琼, 张燕萍, 樊茂蓉. (2012) 加味止嗽散治疗 28 例咳嗽变异性哮喘. 中国实验方剂学杂志 **18(05):** 227–230.
H74	欧阳晓平, 吴峰, 顾扬, 陶玉坚, 黄玉民. (2013) 沙美特罗替卡松联合苏黄止咳胶囊治疗咳嗽变异性哮喘疗效观察. 临床肺科杂志 **18(02):** 257–258.
H75	潘熠. (2015) 宁风理肺汤治疗肝火犯肺型咳嗽变异型哮喘的临床疗效观察. 北京中医药大学.
H76	彭曒, 周荣. (2007) 抗变止嗽汤治疗咳嗽变异型哮喘 57 例. 四川中医. **25(07):** 67–68.

(*Continued*)

(Continued)

Study No.	Reference
H77	浦明之. (2010) 定喘汤合舒利迭治疗咳嗽变异性哮喘 50 例总结. 湖南中医杂志 **26(02)**: 25–26.
H78	齐密霞, 杨艳芳, 宋娟, 贺敬波. (2014) 自拟麻杏汤治疗变异性哮喘慢性咳嗽疗效观察. 现代中西医结合杂志 **23(16)**: 1774–1776.
H79	齐文龙. (2013) 潜龙止咳汤治疗咳嗽变异性哮喘 (肝阳偏亢, 肺气不清证) 的临床观察. 长春中医药大学.
H80	祁海燕. (2009) 润肺止咳法治疗咳嗽变异性哮喘的临床和实验研究. 中国中医科学院.
H81	秦文. (2016) 加减柴胡枳桔汤对咳嗽变异性哮喘患者血清 IL-12, 总 IgE的影响及临床疗效观察. 云南中医学院.
H82	屈毓敏, 王雪京. (2014) 疏风解痉法联合西药治疗 52 例咳嗽变异性哮喘临床观察. 中国医药导报 **11(13)**: 92–95.
H83	曲妮妮, 马智. (2006) 马智教授应用加减止嗽散治疗咳嗽变异性哮喘经验. 中医药学刊 **24(02)**: 212–213.
H84	任先杰, 廖德英, 陈东. (2015) 苏黄止咳胶囊辅助治疗咳嗽变异性哮喘的临床疗效. 临床合理用药杂志 **8(33)**: 127–128.
H85	宋莉. (2014) 咳嗽 2 号方治疗痰热夹风型咳嗽变异性哮喘的疗效观察. 福建中医药大学.
H86	苏利生, 蔡建群, 陈泽滨. (2015) 麻杏苡甘汤化裁辨治湿热郁肺证咳嗽变异性哮喘的临床研究. 中医临床研究 **7(08)**: 74–76.
H87	孙昉, 夏露, 田正鉴. (2009) 疏风固本解痉汤辅助治疗咳嗽变异性哮喘的临床观察. 湖北中医杂志 **31(04)**: 32–33.
H88	孙航成. (2016) 养阴祛风法治疗咳嗽变异性哮喘的临床研究. 南京中医药大学.
H89	孙云晖, 王一新, 马雪梅. (2017) 苏黄止咳胶囊治疗咳嗽变异性哮喘临床研究. 微量元素与健康研究 **34(06)**: 7–9.
H90	覃敏. (2017) 小青花汤加减对咳嗽异性哮喘肺功能的影响研究. 四川中医. **35(5)**: 89–91.
H91	谭家亮. (2015) 自拟慢咳灵方治疗咳嗽变异型哮喘临床疗效观察. 广州中医药大学.
H92	汤俊起, 彭素岚, 敖素华, 王俊峰, 易琳琳, 唐胜. (2011) 清热化痰法治疗咳嗽变异性哮喘 30 例. 河南中医 **31(10)**: 1130–1132.

(Continued)

Study No.	Reference
H93	唐百冬, 何军锋. (2009) 补肾宣肺方治疗肾阳虚咳嗽变异性哮喘临床研究. 中国中医药信息杂志 **16(03):** 12–13.
H94	陶红卫, 姜洪玉. (2008) 血府逐瘀汤加减治疗咳嗽变异性哮喘 50 例疗效观察. 山西中医 **24(09):** 16–17.
H95	滕超. (2017) 止咳平喘汤对咳嗽变异性哮喘 (风盛挛急证) 的临床观察及对血清中 EOS, IL-10 的影响. 黑龙江中医药大学.
H96	王爱皎. (2016) 苏黄止咳胶囊联合布地奈德治疗咳嗽变异性哮喘疗效观察. 人民军医 **59(06):** 582–584.
H97	王东, 杨欣燐, 田琳娟, 张东岳. (2017) 苏黄止咳汤对咳嗽变异性哮喘患者 IL-6, TNF-α 的影响. 中国实验方剂学杂志 **23(02):** 164–168.
H98	王红珊, 李国豪, 曹毅敏, 林美仪, 邓丽丽, 关爱萍. (2012) 射干麻黄汤联合孟鲁司特治疗咳嗽变异型哮喘 86 例. 中国实验方剂学杂志 **18(15):** 273–275.
H99	王军, 丁婷. (2013) 小青龙汤加减合孟鲁司特治疗咳嗽变异性哮喘临床疗效观察. 中国保健营养 (中旬刊) **8(8):** 476.
H100	王宁, 霍晓颖, 陈葆青, 等. (2017) 苏黄止咳胶囊联合舒利迭对咳嗽变异性哮喘患者血清 TNF-α, TGF-β1 和 IgE 水平的影响. 现代生物医学进展 **17(27):** 5298–5301, 5326.
H101	王谦. (2017) 祛风宣肺方治疗 CVA 的疗效观察及其对气道神经源性炎症调控作用的研究. 北京中医药大学.
H102	王秋林. (2014) 加味温胆汤治疗风夹痰热型咳嗽变异性哮喘临床观察. 福建中医药大学.
H103	魏鹏草. (2011) 分型辨证论治咳嗽变异性哮喘临床研究. 北京中医药大学.
H104	吴志宏. (2016) 补益宗气法治疗咳嗽变异性哮喘临床疗效观察. 四川中医 **34(08):** 179–180.
H105	夏露. (2009) 止咳定喘汤治疗咳嗽变异性哮喘 60 例临床分析. 湖北中医学院.
H106	冼峰. (2014) 止嗽散加味治疗咳嗽变异性哮喘 43 例临床观察. 中医药导报 **20(03):** 95–96.
H107	向燕. (2017) 中西医结合治疗咳嗽变异性哮喘的疗效. 世界临床医学 **11(23):** 29.
H108	肖皓明, 王祥生. (2013) 止咳胶囊治疗咳嗽变异型哮喘 30 例. 中国中医药科技 **20(05):** 549–550.

(Continued)

(*Continued*)

Study No.	Reference
H109	谢民栋. (2013) 滋阴清热法治疗咳嗽变异性哮喘随机对照研究. 吉林中医药 **33(02):** 154–155.
H110	辛大永. (2010) 自拟疏肝平嗽汤治疗咳嗽变异性哮喘 31 例. 中国中医药信息杂志 **17(05):** 74.
H111	辛大永. (2015) 九仙散加减治疗咳嗽变异性哮喘的临床观察. 中医药信息 **32(01):** 97–99.
H112	熊艳云. (2011) 培土肃金法治疗痰湿壅肺型咳嗽变异性哮喘的临床观察. 广州中医药大学.
H113	徐常丽. (2014) 自拟养阴清肺方治疗咳嗽变异性哮喘33例临床观察. 中医药导报 **20(04):** 28–29.
H114	徐萍利, 李自力. (2016) 制风止咳汤治疗咳嗽变异性哮喘的疗效分析. 中国中医急症 **25(11):** 2145–2147.
H115	徐启涛, 王东旭, 杨艳玲, 朱琳, 蔡云海. (2014) 清肺止咳汤治疗咳嗽变异性哮喘 40 例. 中医研究 **27(08):** 19–21.
H116	徐伟刚, 钱振萍, 潘敏. (2014) 苏黄止咳胶囊联合复方甲氧那明治疗咳嗽变异性哮喘临床观察. 新中医 **46(01):** 54–56.
H117	许光兰. (2002) 十味龙胆花颗粒治疗咳嗽变异型哮喘 63 例. 中国中医药信息杂志 **9(1):** 72.
H118	薛晓明, 王洋, 赵勤萍, 关炜. (2010) 疏肝祛风止咳方联合普米克都保治疗咳嗽变异性哮喘疗效观察. 新中医 **42(06):** 87–88.
H119	严淑, 王伟平. (2014) 止嗽散加味联合西药治疗咳嗽变异性哮喘疗效观察. 实用中医药杂志 **30(07):** 633–634.
H120	剡雄, 王琦. (2017) 益气祛风方治疗咳嗽变异性哮喘临床观察. 中国中医药信息杂志. **24(11):** 30–33.
H121	杨慧敏, 张超, 王倩倩. (2017) 麻杏祛风颗粒治疗咳嗽变异性哮喘随机对照试验. 临床医药文献电子杂志 **4(27):** 5292–5293.
H122	杨舒雅, 孟泳, 甘德堃. (2017) 加味过敏煎辅助治疗咳嗽变异性哮喘 30 例. 中国中医药现代远程教育 **15(20):** 97–98.
H123	杨树升, 林丽, 向艳丽. (2012) 小青龙汤治疗咳嗽变异性哮喘的临床疗效分析. 现代医药卫生 **28(06):** 901–903.
H124	杨毅勇, 陈晓宏. (2015) 调肝肃肺汤治疗咳嗽变异性哮喘临床观察. 上海中医药大学学报. **29(01):**30-32+36.

(Continued)

Study No.	Reference
H125	叶丹丹, 毛敏华. (2015) 加味三拗汤联合孟鲁司特钠片治疗咳嗽变异性哮喘疗效观察. 新中医 **47(07):** 48–50.
H126	叶焰, 金华伟, 里自然. (2015) 健脾肃肺法对痰湿蕴肺型咳嗽变异性哮喘患者生活质量的影响. 吉林医学 **36(10):** 2096.
H127	叶焰, 熊艳云. (2013) 健脾肃肺法治疗痰湿蕴肺型 CVA 的临床观察. 医学信息 **26(5):** 236–237.
H128	游伟玲, 李晓珍, 张锋, 刘胜. (2017) 中西医结合治疗咳嗽变异性哮喘临床观察. 新中医. **49(06):** 40–42.
H129	余静. (2016) 祛风宣肺法治疗风痰阻肺型咳嗽变异性哮喘的临床研究. 南京中医药大学.
H130	余晓琪, 干磊, 程德华. (2011) 润燥祛风法治疗咳嗽变异性哮喘的随机对照研究. 上海中医药杂志 **45(05):** 58–59.
H131	袁安冬, 李红涛. (2007) 过敏煎合二陈汤治疗咳嗽变异型哮喘和对血清 IgE 值的影响. 光明中医 **22(07):** 53–54.
H132	张芬. (2014) 华盖散加味汤治疗咳嗽变异性哮喘 (风盛挛急证) 的临床疗效研究. 成都中医药大学.
H133	张桂才, 仇中叶, 蔡元培, 林敏, 孙洪林, 乐进. (2013) 固本止咳颗粒治疗咳嗽变异性哮喘临床研究. 中国中医药信息杂志 **20(12):** 9–11.
H134	张杰. (2017) 苏黄止咳胶囊治疗咳嗽变异型哮喘临床观察. 河南中医 **37(09):** 1604–1606.
H135	张群. (2013) 三三九咳散治疗咳嗽变异性哮喘 51 例临床研究. 中国中医急症 **22(06):** 909–911.
H136	张群, 陈继忠, 孙学会, 等. (2011) 止嗽散加味颗粒剂联合信必可治疗咳嗽变异性哮喘的临床研究. 国际中医中药杂志 **33(6):** 487–490.
H137	张蓉, 吴昆仑. (2012) 自拟抗敏止咳方治疗咳嗽变异型哮喘 42 例. 上海中医药杂志 **46(05):** 53–54.
H138	张伟. (2011) 晁恩祥教授诊治"风咳"临床应用评价研究. 广州中医药大学.
H139	张亚萍. (2016) 中西结合治疗咳嗽变异性哮喘 (风痰证) 的临床研究. 南京中医药大学.
H140	张彦峰. (2008) 逍遥散治疗咳嗽变异型哮喘 (肝郁脾虚, 肺气上逆) 临床研究. 长春中医药大学.

(Continued)

(Continued)

Study No.	Reference
H141	张颖, 刘雪晴, 伍彩霞, 张小丹. (2006) 止咳抗敏汤治疗咳嗽变异型哮喘 45 例. 上海中医药杂志 **40(6):** 23–24.
H142	章福宝, 陶怡, 宁静. (2015) 止咳方联合西医治疗咳嗽变异性哮喘临床观察. 新中医 **47(03):** 60–62.
H143	章海峰, 沈佩雷. (2015) 苏黄止咳胶囊联合阿斯美治疗咳嗽变异型哮喘 80 例临床观察. 中国医学创新 **12(10):** 34–37.
H144	赵柏庆, 林秀云, 尹海燕, 林宏超, 梁文华. (2015) 人参蛤蚧散合止嗽散对咳嗽变异性哮喘疗效探讨. 光明中医 **30(11):** 2327–2329.
H145	赵红霞, 冯海军. (2015) 益气补肾汤联合沙美特罗替卡松治疗咳嗽变异性哮喘的临床观察. 中国医药导刊 **17(03):** 282–283.
H146	支艳, 杨明会, 张印, 刘毅, 赵宏. (2011) 滋阴清热补肺益肾法治疗咳嗽变异性哮喘的临床研究. 中医临床研究 **3(5):** 1–3.
H147	支艳, 赵宏, 曹璐. (2009) 滋阴清热法治疗咳嗽变异性哮喘临床研究. 中国中医急症 **18(12):** 1956–1958.
H148	钟丹. (2014) 中药敏咳煎对阴虚肺燥型CVA患者气道神经源性炎症影响及生活质量干预研究. 成都中医药大学.
H149	钟云青. (2017) 宣肺止嗽合剂辅助治疗咳嗽变异性哮喘的风邪犯肺证患者. 中成药 **39(05):** 912–915.
H150	周宝银, 张静, 张爱观, 刘吕敏, 陈坤, 何卉, *et al.* (2016) 桃红止嗽散联合舒利迭对咳嗽变异性哮喘患者肺功能的影响. 中国中医药科技 **23(02):** 189–190.
H151	周勤. (2014) 中西医结合治疗对咳嗽变异型哮喘患者肺功能的影响. 内科 **9(1):** 6–8.
H152	朱金凤, 陈梅玲, 彭俊杰, 李卫青, 柯新桥. (2006) 固本平喘汤治疗咳嗽变异型哮喘的临床观察. 湖北中医杂志 **28(8):** 12–14.
H153	朱琳. (2015) 十二味止咳合剂联合舒利迭治疗咳嗽变异性哮喘60例临床观察. 云南中医中药杂志 **36(02):** 28–29.
H154	朱文静. (2015) 苏黄止咳胶囊辅助治疗咳嗽变异性哮喘的临床研究. 药物评价研究 **38(03):** 310–313.
H155	朱筱慧, 林云辉, 赵慧霞, 于世杰, 张连霞, 康千宽, *et al.* (2016) 应用苏黄止咳胶囊联合信必可吸入治疗咳嗽变异性哮喘 (CVA) 的疗效及安全性. 中国医药指南 **14(34):** 159–160.
H156	朱迎霞, 李金润. (2013) 苏黄止咳胶囊联合西药治疗咳嗽变异型哮喘 25 例临床观察. 云南中医中药杂志 **34(3):** 23–24, 89.

(*Continued*)

Study No.	Reference
H157	卓进盛. (2012) 加味止嗽散治疗咳嗽变异型哮喘. 中国实验方剂学杂志 **18(1)**: 217–219.
H158	陈伦, 祁佳, 张宇锋. (2015) 黄芪颗粒治疗咳嗽变异性哮喘临床研究. 现代中西医结合杂志 **24(15)**: 1597–1599.
H159	蓝杨, 张海艇. (2015) 孟鲁司特联合止咳中成药治疗咳嗽变异性哮喘的临床观察. 世界临床医学 **9(11)**: 172–173.
H160	卢世秀, 李步满, 尹李虎, 向平超, 张二明, 王雪京, *et al.* (2016) 疏风止嗽方治疗咳嗽变异性哮喘临床研究. 中国中医药信息杂志 **23(12)**: 30–33.
H161	卢世秀, 尹李虎, 李步满, 向平超, 张二明, 王雪京, *et al.* (2017) 调中益肺方联合西药治疗咳嗽变异性哮喘缓解期临床观察. 中国中医药信息杂志 **24(7)**: 36–39.
H162	邱容, 肖昌武, 文富强. (2017) 布地奈德福莫特罗联合苏黄止咳胶囊对咳嗽变异性哮喘的疗效观察. 临床肺科杂志 **22(2)**: 304–306.
H163	吴青青. (2015) 抗敏止嗽颗粒治疗CVA的临床疗效及对呼出气一氧化氮水平的影响. 河南中医学院.
H164	张爱平, 黄龙, 郑玉琼, 黄建果, 尹洁, 李洪成, *et al.* (2011) 中西医结合治疗对尘螨过敏的咳嗽变异型哮喘患者肺功能及1年复发率的影响. 新中医 **43(8)**: 10–11.
H165	郑玉琼, 张爱平, 黄龙, 黄建果, 尹洁, 李洪成. (2010) 中西医联合方案治疗咳嗽变异性哮喘的疗效评估. 四川中医 **28(9)**: 58–60.
H166	卓致远. (2014) 布地奈德福莫特罗粉吸入剂联合苏黄止咳胶囊治疗咳嗽变异性哮喘的临床疗效观察. 实用心脑肺血管病杂志 **22(12)**: 91–92.
H167	马嘉蓉, 张春霞, 韩玉, 巴迎莹, 刘淑芸. (2017) 布地奈德福莫特罗粉吸入剂联合中医药辨证治疗老年咳嗽变异性哮喘. 重庆医学 **46(21)**: 2962–2965.
H168	严建雄, 麦妙坚, 谭子珍. (2017) 探讨疏风通络方治疗风痰型咳嗽变异性哮喘的效果. 内蒙古中医药 **36(Z1)**: 10–11.
H169	张彦峰. (2017) 疏风止咳散治疗咳嗽变异性哮喘风邪犯肺型 72 例临床疗效观察. 中国保健营养 **17(6)**: 407
H170	张杨, 刘若实, 张杰. (2015) 止嗽散加减联合万托林气雾剂治疗咳嗽变异性哮喘临床观察. 中国医师杂志 **17(5)**: 748–749.
H171	张佑, 吴双. (2017) 孟鲁司特钠联合苏黄止咳胶囊治疗咳嗽变异性哮喘的临床疗效及安全性研究. 山西医药杂志 **46(16)**: 1990–1992.

(*Continued*)

(Continued)

Study No.	Reference
H172	宗喜中, 成爱武. (2014) 中西医结合治疗咳嗽变异性哮喘50例. 中国中医药现代远程教育. **12(24):** 61–62.
H173	方灵云. (2011) 射干麻黄汤加味治疗咳嗽变异性哮喘(寒咳型) 43 例疗效观察. 浙江中医药大学学报 **35(03):** 336–337.
H174	李光, 王敏. (2010) 宣肺止嗽汤治疗咳嗽变异性哮喘 134 例. 山西中医 **26(2):** 16.
H175	林朝亮, 蔡元培, 张桂才. (2010) 风咳汤加减治疗咳嗽变异性哮喘 47 例. 光明中医 **25(12):** 2224–2225.
H176	谢嘉嘉, 梁建华, 彭俊杰, 曾小玲, 林国彬. (2012) 基于 IL-13, NF-Kb p65 变化探讨小青龙汤干预咳嗽变异性哮喘临床研究. 中医学报 **27(11):** 1398–1400.
H177	谢纬. (2010) 小青龙汤加味治疗咳嗽变异性哮喘(寒咳型) 38 例疗效观察. 新中医 **42(10):** 19–20.
H178	张峰, 钱静华. (2007) 止嗽散加味治疗咳嗽变异性哮喘 40 例. 吉林中医药 **27(11):** 33.
H179	张业清, 朱启勇, 黄雅菊, 孙航成, 肖庆铃, 李朝娟, *et al.* (2013) 宣肺平喘方治疗咳嗽变异性哮喘的有效性和对 FeNO 影响临床研究. 辽宁中医杂志 **40(12):** 2504–2506.
H180	左冬冬, 滕林, 李兰. (2015) 宣肺化痰平喘止咳法治疗变异性哮喘的临床观察. 中医药信息 **32(03):** 110–112.
H181	陈瑞琳, 杨珺超, 王真. (2015) 疏风通窍法治疗上气道咳嗽综合征 32 例临床观察. 浙江中医杂志 **50(07):** 493.
H182	何宛芸, 卢云. (2017) 麻黄细辛附子汤加味治疗上气道咳嗽综合征的临床观察. 中国民族民间医药 **26(1):** 103–106.
H183	李敏芳, 李亚清, 陈生, 熊广, 谢纬. (2015) 上气道咳嗽方治疗上气道咳嗽综合征的临床观察. 内蒙古中医药 **34(7):** 14–15.
H184	刘洁华, 郭永坚. (2012) 自拟疏风通窍利咽汤治疗上气道咳嗽综合征 36 例. 中国民间疗法 **20(1):** 34–35.
H185	刘英文, 陈柏竹. (2016) 中西医结合在气道咳嗽综合征患者中的应用及对肺功能的影响研究. 中国现代医生 **54(31):** 18–21.
H186	吕天璞. (2012) 疏风宣肺、化痰利咽法治疗上气道咳嗽综合征（风痰恋肺证）的临床研究. 南京中医药大学.
H187	秦莹, 张思文, 顾炳岐. (2010) 中药内外同治法治疗鼻后滴流综合征致慢性咳嗽的临床研究. 上海中医药杂志 **44(5):** 57–59.

(Continued)

Study No.	Reference
H188	史锁芳, 魏瑜, 王德钧, 谈欧, 徐静, 朱际平, *et al.* (2010) 疏风宣肺、化痰利咽法治疗上气道咳嗽综合征52例临床观察. 江苏中医药 **42(12)**: 30–31.
H189	史锁芳, 张念志, 万丽玲, 邹建东, 陈宝华, 苏强, *et al.* (2013) 疏风宣肺化痰利咽方为主治疗上气道咳嗽综合征 195 例临床观察. 中医杂志 **54(7)**: 576–579.
H190	王蓓娟. (2014) 宣肺清热利咽方治疗上气道咳嗽综合征 43 例疗效分析. 中外医疗. **33(33)**: 146–150.
H191	杨莉惠. (2011) 加味咳平汤治疗风邪犯肺型上气道咳嗽综合征临床观察. 福建中医药大学.
H192	刘淑芸. (2016) 小柴胡汤加减治疗上气道咳嗽综合征的临床研究. 西南医科大学.
H193	郝小梅, 孙珍, 刘梅. (2014) 疏风利咽止咳汤治疗上气道咳嗽综合征 58 例疗效观察. 新中医 **46(5)**: 56–57.
H194	李光, 陈昆, 王春雨. (2011) 温肺止流丹加味治疗上气道咳嗽综合征 40 例. 河南中医 **31(1)**: 56.
H195	车彦贞. (2017) 半夏厚朴汤治疗胃食管反流性咳嗽临床观察. 中国民族民间医药 **26(20)**: 89–90.
H196	桯序, 廖成荣, 李东方, 赵彦祺, 陈小会. (2017) 安胃止嗽煎治疗胃食管反流性咳嗽临床观察. 实用中医药杂志 **33(8)**: 908–909.
H197	丁明升. (2012) 辛开苦降法治疗胃咳的临床观察. 山东中医药大学.
H198	冯超. (2017) 中药四逆散加味治疗胃食管反流性咳嗽的疗效. 临床与病理杂志 **37(7)**: 1423–1428.
H199	符滨, 杨艳娜, 刘敏. (2014) 中西药结合治疗胃食管反流性咳嗽临床疗效观察. 亚太传统医药 **10(20)**: 47–49.
H200	高伟, 马利荣, 陈敏华, 钟巍, 孙庆琴, 李雨, *et al.* (2017) 自拟疏木运土止咳方结合西医常规疗法治疗胃食管反流性咳嗽临床研究. 国际中医中药杂志 **39**(5): 420–423.
H201	关妙连. (2014) 中医结合健康宣教治疗胃食管反流性咳嗽的临床观察. 广州中医药大学.
H202	何志良. (2008) 四逆散加味治疗胃食管反流性咳嗽临床观察. 中华实用中西医杂志 **21(15)**: 1255–1256.
H203	李光, 陈锐, 孟文媛, 徐莺, 吕蒙, 范娟娟. (2014) 和胃降逆法治疗胃食管反流性咳嗽临床观察. 山西中医 **30(6)**: 9–12.

(Continued)

(*Continued*)

Study No.	Reference
H204	刘春芳, 郭召平, 曹会杰, 程艳梅, 张秀莲, 朱生樑, *et al.* (2013) 通降和胃方治疗胃食管反流性咳嗽 60 例. 环球中医药 **6(7):** 539–541.
H205	潘业明. (2014) 和胃止咳汤治疗胃食管反流性咳嗽（肝胃不和型）的临床研究. 长春中医药大学.
H206	王北辰. (2015) 半夏泻心汤加减联合质子泵抑制剂治疗胃食管反流性咳嗽的临床观察. 中国现代药物应用 **9(7):** 156–158.
H207	夏迪娅, 夏木西丁, 于碧馨, 段红霞. (2015) 温胃降逆颗粒联合质子泵抑制剂治疗胃食管反流性咳嗽的疗效观察. 中医药导报 **21(17):** 65–67.
H208	张天涛, 宋玉勤, 侯宝松, 刘霞, 田国芳. (2016) 四逆散加减对胃食管反流性咳嗽患者诱导痰细胞及相关介质水平的影响. 河北中医 **38(6):** 891–895.
H209	张瑛. (2013) 和胃温胆汤治疗胃食管反流性咳嗽 35 例观察. 浙江中医杂志 **48(10):** 724.
H210	赵丽芸, 陈宁. (2011) 加味半夏厚朴汤治疗胃食管反流性咳嗽38例临床观察. 中医药导报 **17(6):** 27–29.
H211	傅遂山. (2011) 中西医结合治疗胃食管反流性咳嗽 38 例. 中医研究 **24(2):** 49–50.
H212	李光, 孟文媛, 尹美凤. (2011) 自拟和胃止嗽汤治疗胃食管反流性咳嗽 48 例疗效观察. 云南中医中药杂志 **32(2):** 40.

6

Pharmacological Actions of Frequently Used Herbs

OVERVIEW

Herbal medicines have therapeutic effects largely attributable to their active compounds. To understand the possible biological activity of the most frequently used herbs in randomised controlled trials, this chapter provides a summary of the experimental evidence and relevant mechanisms of action related to the pathophysiological processes of chronic cough.

Introduction

Chinese herbs and their constituent compounds exert various pharmacological effects. Experimental evidence including *in vitro* and *in vivo* studies help to explain the possible mechanisms of action of the herbs and how they may improve the signs and symptoms of chronic cough. This chapter examines the pharmacological actions of the top ten herbs identified in randomised controlled trials (RCTs) by identifying experimental cellular processes and animal models for chronic cough. The evidence provides biological plausibility and possible explanations for the positive benefits identified in clinical trials.

The mechanisms of cough are complex, and the pathogenesis differs depending on the cough type and stimuli. There are some overlapping mechanisms, such as sensitisation of the cough reflex, but there are also unique elements depending on the type, such as cough variant asthma (CVA), upper airways cough syndrome (UACS) or gastro-oesophageal reflux disease (GORD). In most cases, airway inflammation and tissue remodelling are present causing an ongoing and enhanced cough reflex.[1] It is therefore important to look for the underlying cause and, if possible, treat the cause to alleviate the cough. However, sometimes it is not possible to find a cause, or the cause cannot be treated, for example post-viral cough, pertussis cough and cough due to pulmonary fibrosis. In these situations, treatments are needed to directly suppress the cough.

Asthma, in which cough is the predominant symptom, is sometimes referred to as CVA. The underlying pathophysiology is still one of airway inflammation, predominantly with eosinophils.[2] This leads to airway hyper-reactivity and bronchospasm, and in some patients may lead to airway remodelling in the long-term. Conventional treatment is with inhaled corticosteroids, often combined with a long-acting beta agonist, to suppress the airway inflammation.

Upper airways cough syndrome, on the other hand, is not a clearly defined disease; rather a syndrome where nasal and sinus secretions drip into the pharynx and larynx stimulating cough receptors. Therefore, pathophysiological processes may vary, including allergic and non-allergic rhinitis, chronic rhinosinusitis, infections or polyps. Inflammation may play a role where inflammatory mediators stimulate cough receptors previously activated by a nervous reflex. These are induced by inflammatory stimulation of nasal mucosa, nasal neural activation and pharyngeal and/or laryngeal neural sensitivity.[3] Treatments for UACS including corticosteroids, antihistamines and anticholinergics give some insight into the pathophysiology of disease.

Chronic cough related to GORD also has a complex mechanism. Acid that refluxes from the stomach into the lower oesophagus causes vagal nerve stimulation and coughing. Reflux micro-aspiration may also directly impact the bronchial tree leading to bronchial hyper-responsiveness. Over time the repetitive cough leads to structural and inflammatory airway changes. It is also thought that reflux causes mechanical and chemical stimulation of cough receptors, and a cough reflex feedback mechanism is activated. Treatments are more holistic and include diet and lifestyle modification, as well as drugs such as proton pump inhibitors to block stomach acid, and others such as alginates to prevent the reflux wave.

To identify experimental studies relevant to chronic cough, the pharmacological activities of each herb were assessed in terms of their therapeutic effects on pulmonary inflammation, antihistamine and anticholinergic actions, as well as prevention of reflux. This is in addition to cough suppression, and bronchial hyper-responsiveness if available. The cough mechanism can be mimicked in animal models including guinea pigs, cats and dogs, but is less reliable in rodents because their cough reflex does not closely resemble humans. The conscious guinea pig cough model is thought to be broadly representative of the human tussive response after stimulation with agents such as capsaicin and citric acid.

Chronic cough mechanisms are more difficult to mimic due to the interplay of peripheral and central mechanisms where, for example, resolution of peripheral inflammation/stimuli may not completely resolve chronic cough. Tissue damage from repeated cough and airway inflammation increases sensory afferent activity producing plasticity in central pathways.[4] This central hyper-responsiveness is not unique to chronic cough but also present in other systems, such as neurogenic pain.[5] Despite some limitations, animal models of cough can be illustrative and provide valuable information about the mechanisms of herbal medicine.

Inflammatory models in macrophages and murine models can also help to understand the mechanisms of the herbs, although they do not exactly reproduce the characteristic features of human inflammation. For example, macrophages (a type of leukocyte) stimulate the immune system and initiate inflammatory responses including inflammatory mediators, such as tumour necrosis factor alpha (TNF-α), interleukin 1beta (IL-1β) and interleukin 6 (IL-6), as well as nitric oxide (NO) and prostaglandin E2 (PGE2).[6] In lipopolysaccharide (LPS) animal models there is a systemic inflammatory response that is relatively easy to measure. Therefore, supressing the inflammatory response in macrophages and LPS-stimulated mice models can illustrate the potential benefits and mechanisms of the actions of the herbs.

The ten most common herbs identified in RCTs (Chapter 5) and therefore evaluated in this chapter are *ma huang* 麻黄, *gan cao* 甘草,

xing ren 杏仁, *chan tui* 蝉蜕, *jie geng* 桔梗, *di long* 地龙, *wu wei zi* 五味子, *zi wan* 紫菀, *ban xia* 半夏 and *zi su ye* 紫苏叶.

Methods

This chapter provides a general overview of the experimental evidence relating to the pharmacology of herbs and their constituent compounds for chronic cough. The constituent compounds were identified by searching herbal monographs, high-quality reviews of Chinese herbal medicine, herbal medicine encyclopedia,[7] materia medica[8] and PubMed. To identify pre-clinical studies, literature searches in PubMed were undertaken. The search strategy included the names of the herb in Chinese *pinyin* and scientific names, and the names of compounds contained in the herbs. These were combined with the terms chronic cough, cough, CVA, UACS, GORD, pulmonary disorders, antitussive, inflammation, allergy and reflux. Relevant data were extracted and a summary of the findings are reported here.

Experimental Studies on *Ma Huang* 麻黄

Ma huang 麻黄 (*Ephedra sinica* Stapf) contains alkaloids such as ephedrine and pseudo-ephedrine, volatile oils and flavonoids.[7,8] Ephedrine is an adrenoceptor agonist that increases norepinephrine release. Therefore, it can stimulate the central nervous system. In addition, *ma huang* 麻黄 has shown anti-inflammatory effects that may be important for the treatment of CVA and UACS. *Ma huang* 麻黄 combined with other herbs in the formula *Ma huang tang* 麻黄汤 has anti-inflammatory effects shown in an asthma mouse model.[9] It also has potent decongestant and bronchodilator effects.

Ma huang 麻黄 has significant vasoconstrictor activity in the pulmonary vascular bed mediated by α1-adrenergic receptor activation.[10] This may be an important mechanism for suppression of cough by interacting with cardiovascular and respiratory neuronal systems and stimulating arterial baroreceptors.[11] It is for this reason that *ma huang* 麻黄 should be used with caution. It has some reported side effects such as high blood pressure, restlessness and insomnia, and is not recommended for long-term use.[12] *Ma huang* 麻黄 is also restricted in some countries, and readers are advised to check local regulations.

Experimental Studies on *Gan Cao* 甘草

Gan cao 甘草 (Licorice root) includes several species in Chinese medicine (CM), most commonly *Glycyrrhiza uralensis* Fisch., *Glycyrrhiza inflata* Bat. and *Glycyrrhiza glabra* L. *Gan cao* 甘草 contains many bioactive constituents including triterpenes (e.g. glycyrrhizic acid or glycyrrhizin), coumarin derivates, alkaloids and various types of flavonoids.[8] The compounds of *gan cao* 甘草 have diverse pharmacological properties, such as anti-inflammatory, anti-oxidative, antiulcerative, antiallergic, antiviral and hepatoprotective, and specifically for cough it is an expectorant.[13]

Antitussive Actions

Gan cao 甘草 and its compounds possess antitussive properties. In guinea pigs *gan cao's* constituent compound, liquiritin apioside (3–30 mg/kg, per oral [p.o.]) and metabolite liquiritigenin reduced capsaicin-induced cough frequency by acting on peripheral receptors in the airway and central receptors in the serotonergic system.[14–16] Isoliquiritigenin also has antispasmodic and analgesic actions in guinea pig tracheal smooth muscle cells.[17] Crude *gan cao* 甘草 extracts and polysaccharides also have antitussive effects shown in cough models of guinea pigs.[16,18,19] In one study, cough was induced by microinjection of citric acid solution into the larynx. Herbs were then given to the guinea pigs in their water for three days. *Gan cao* 甘草 significantly reduced cough frequency, similar to codeine (a known cough suppressant control). The mechanism of actions is likely through central antitussive effects[20] and/or stimulation of β2-adrenoceptors that relax tracheal smooth muscle and bronchial passages to reduce cough.[21]

Anti-inflammatory Actions

Gan cao 甘草 compounds have anti-inflammatory properties likely related to their mineralocorticoid action.[22] In an asthma model using

161

ovalbumin (OVA)-sensitised mice, glycyrrhizinic acid reduced airway resistance and suppressed the generation of a type 2 helper T cell (Th2)-type immune response.[23] Furthermore, 7,4'-dihydroxyflavone (DHF) also reduced eosinophilic pulmonary inflammation in lung cell cultures.[24] Glycyrrhizin and licochalcone A, compounds found in *gan cao* 甘草, can reduce inflammatory cell recruitment including eosinophils, neutrophils, lymphocytes and macrophages, as well as inhibit cytokines in bronchoalveolar lavage fluid (BALF) in allergic asthmatic mice.[25,26]

Antiallergic Actions

In UACS and CVA, allergic causes are common. Glycyrrhizic and glycyrrhetic acids regulate immune cells and have antiallergic effects, possibly due to its ability to antagonise H_1-histamine receptors.[22] There are a large number of studies that indicate it can significantly reduce allergic reactions, which is an important component of CVA. In allergic asthma models, the compounds glycyrrhizin, licochalcone A and 7,4'-DHF (all derived from *gan cao* 甘草) inhibited Th2 cytokines in BALF, reduced immunoglobulin type E and G (IgE and IgG, respectively), and reduced eosinophil, neutrophil, lymphocyte and macrophage inflammatory cell recruitment.[24–26] In an OVA-induced mouse model, *gan cao* 甘草 reduced allergic symptoms in line with hydrocortisone, regulated the expression of Th1 and Th2 cytokines, and reduced allergic responses.[27] The flavonoids isoliquiritigenin, 7,4'-DHF and liquiritigenin flavonoids reduced allergic reactions by suppressing cytokine production (IL-4 and IL-5) and cell proliferation in Th2 D10 cells. Taken together, these studies indicate that *gan cao* 甘草 can have a significant impact on allergic and inflammatory aspects of chronic cough, especially when used for CVA.

Antireflux Actions

In some cases, people with GORD can benefit from improved gastric motility. Gastric acid secretions can increase when there is prolonged exposure of material in the stomach. A flavonoid isolated from *gan cao* 甘草 (isoliquiritigenin) can regulate gastrointestinal motility and improve digestive function.[28] In another study, a commercial formulation of *Glycyrrhiza inflate* demonstrated gastroprotective and gastric motility benefits by speeding up gastric emptying in rats.[29] Glycyrrhizin has been studied for its effect on ulcer healing. It can reduce inflammatory mediators and regulate amino acid metabolism, and effectively treat gastric ulcers in mice.[30] Although it is not a direct effect on reflux or cough, these results indicate important gastrointestinal actions that might be important in reducing GORD and in turn reducing cough.

Experimental Studies on *Xing Ren* 杏仁

Xing ren 杏仁 (*Prunus armeniaca* L. var. *ansu* Maxim.) contains several bioactive compounds including glycosides, amygdalin, amygdalase and oils such as oleic acid and linoleic acid.[7,8] It has a long history of use in CM for inflammatory conditions of the lungs, stomach and skin, but most commonly it is used for cough. Experimental studies have shown antioxidant, antimicrobial and antitussive effects. Due to the presence of cyanogenic glycosides in *xing ren* 杏仁, the therapeutic application and dose need to be monitored to avoid toxic effects.[31]

Antitussive Actions

In a cough model in mice, the *xing ren* 杏仁 compound amygdalin had antitussive effects. Sulfur dioxide gas was used to induce cough and amygdalin (1.0, 10 and 100 mg/kg p.o.) inhibited cough induction.[32] More recent studies have assessed the antitussive effects of *xing ren* 杏仁 combined with other herbs. *Xing ren* 杏仁, *ma huang* 麻黄, *gan cao* 甘草 and shi gao 石膏 were evaluated in citric acid-induced cough and acetylcholine/histamine-induced bronchial contraction in guinea pigs.[33] The herbs (administered for 28 days) produced significant dose-dependent antitussive effects and blocked bronchial contraction induced by acetylcholine/histamine.

Anti-inflammatory Actions

Xing ren 杏仁 can reduce oxidative damage and apoptosis in rats stimulated with methotrexate.[34] A study assessing antimicrobial activities of an oil derived from *xing ren* 杏仁 showed a reduction in gram-positive and gram-negative bacteria and yeasts. The *xing ren* 杏仁 extracts also scavenged free radicals and inhibited lipid peroxidation *in vitro*.[35,36]

Xing ren 杏仁, combined with other herbs, has been studied in several pulmonary inflammation models. In a cockroach allergen-induced asthma model, the number of leukocytes, eosinophils, neutrophils, lymphocytes and macrophages was reduced in BALF.[37] To further elucidate the benefits, lung tissue damage and inflammatory cell infiltration into the airways was also observed. The *xing ren* 杏仁 herb combination reduced inflammatory cells in the peribronchial regions, demonstrating its potential benefit to reduce lung tissue damage. In another asthma model in rats, a *xing ren* 杏仁 herb combination alleviated pulmonary inflammatory pathological damage and downregulated inflammatory cell and mediator infiltration in pulmonary tissues.[38] In a chronic obstructive pulmonary disease (COPD) model, the same combination of herbs also attenuated lung inflammation by reducing airway hyper-responsiveness and immune cells in BALF.[39] Despite studies not being conducted in CVA, UACS or GORD models, the results may have implications for these conditions as there is a significant inflammatory response and link between chronic cough and pulmonary inflammation.

Antiallergic Actions

In a murine allergic airway inflammation model, *xing ren* 杏仁 combined with other herbs reduced the production of inflammatory mediators such as IgE and the Th2 type immune response.[37] The Th2 cytokines and allergic response mediators decreased, as did proinflammatory functions. In a mouse model of allergic asthma, a crude extract of *xing ren* 杏仁 reduced airway hyper-reactivity, indicating suppression of the Th2 response, and in turn reducing allergic asthma-induced airway inflammation.[40]

Experimental Studies on *Chan Tui* 蝉蜕

Chan tui 蝉蜕 is derived from Cicada slough *(Cryptotympana pustulata* Fabricius). The major active compounds are chitin and several amino acids such as alanin, proline and aspartic acid.[8] Despite its broad use for respiratory and throat conditions, there are only a few studies evaluating its mechanisms of action for cough. The antitussive, phlegm-resolving and anti-asthmatic effects of *chan tui* 蝉蜕 and its active ingredients in animals have been evaluated. *Chan tui* 蝉蜕 decoction can reduce cough induced by inhalation of ammonia by prolonging the duration to cough onset in mice. It can also increase phenol red excretion in the trachea of mice and prolong the duration to acetylcholine and histamine-induced asthma onset in guinea pigs.[41,42] The water fraction is the active part relevant to cough; n-butanol is the active compound relevant to reducing sputum; and the water fraction and ethyl acetate extract are active parts for relieving asthma.[41]

Chan tui 蝉蜕 has a range of antioxidative and anti-inflammatory actions. The *Cryptotympana atrata* species was evaluated for its anti-inflammatory effects in mice with contact dermatitis.[43] It inhibited immune cell infiltration and supressed TNF-α, IFN-gamma and IL-6 production. Although the results relate to inflammatory skin disease, future research will help to elucidate its effects in pulmonary inflammation.

Experimental Studies on *Jie Geng* 桔梗

Jie geng 桔梗 species, *Platycodon grandiflorus* (Jacq.) A.DC., contains many bioactive compounds such as triterpene saponin glycosides (platycodin, polygalacin), sapogenines (polycodigenin and polygalacic acid), prosapogenines, polysaccharides (platycodinin) and phytosteroils. In traditional CM it is used for cough, excessive phlegm and sore throat.[44]

Antitussive Actions

Jie geng 桔梗 decoction can inhibit cough induced by ammonia by prolonging the cough incubation period in mice.[45] After 30 days, *jie geng* 桔梗 decoction at 1.3 g/kg, 2.6 g/kg and 5.4 g/kg reduced the total number of leukocytes in lung tissue. *Jie geng* 桔梗 also decreased the cough frequency in histamine-induced asthma and citric acid-induced cough models.[45] *Jie geng* 桔梗 is also an expectorant that can increase sputum/mucus, in turn improving airway respiratory function and preventing secondary airway inflammation.[46] In sulfur dioxide-induced bronchitis in rats, an aqueous extract of *jie geng* 桔梗 significantly increased airway mucin.[47] Its constituent compounds, the triterpenoid saponins platycodin D and D3, also increased airway mucin in rats, hamsters and airway epithelial cells.[46]

Anti-inflammatory Actions

Jie geng 桔梗 and its active constituents have been extensively studied *in vitro* and *in vivo* for their anti-inflammatory effects.[44] Beta-sitosterol found in *jie geng* 桔梗 can attenuate pulmonary fibrosis[48] whereas botulin and platycodin D can reduce cigarette smoke-induced lung inflammation in mice,[49,50] and crude extracts can inhibit inflammatory pathways and genes in human cultured airway epithelial cells.[51] In acute and chronic lung inflammation mouse models, intraperitoneal platycodin D for five days attenuated lung pathological changes and inflammatory cell infiltration, as well as TNF-α and IL-1β production.[50] After eight weeks of intragastric botulin (20mg/kg and 40mg/kg), pathological injury in lung tissue, as well oxidative stress, were reduced and proinflammatory cytokines were inhibited (TNF-α, IL-6 and IL-1β).[49]

Antiallergic Actions

Ovalbumin-induced airway inflammation in mice was inhibited by *jie geng* 桔梗 root-derived saponins; the results indicated that total saponins, especially platyconic acid A, reduced allergic responses by suppressing respiratory inflammation, hyper-responsiveness and remodelling. The authors indicated that *jie geng* 桔梗 saponins may be suitable for allergen-induced respiratory disease prevention.[52] In a murine chronic airway inflammation asthma model, an aqueous extract of *jie geng* 桔梗 (50 mg/kg) inhibited airway inflammation, leukocyte recruitment and levels of Th1 and Th2 cytokines, IgE and monocyte chemoattractant protein-1 (MCP-1, a chemokine) in the lungs.[52]

Experimental Studies on *Di Long* 地龙

Di long 地龙 is an animal product (earthworm, *Pheretima spp.*) composed of amino acids, xanthines and lipids.[8] It has a long history of use for respiratory and inflammatory diseases such as asthma, cough and fever.

Antitussive Actions

Asthma animal models have shown that *di long* 地龙 fractions reduce histamine-induced contraction of the trachea and cough frequency.[53] Relevant for CVA, xanthines are commonly used for asthma and xanthine drugs have been developed from plants in the past.[54] Xanthines can prevent the release of inflammatory chemicals (e.g. histamine) and stabilise mast cells, therefore reducing inflammation and preventing asthma attacks. To date there are no published experimental studies evaluating the xanthines from *di long* 地龙, but they may be an important compound that helps to exert *di long's* therapeutic effects.

Anti-inflammatory Actions

The effects of *di long* 地龙 were evaluated in RAW 264.7 macrophages stimulated with LPS to trigger an inflammatory response. *Di long* 地龙 at concentrations of 40–320 μg/mL showed broad anti-inflammatory effects by inhibiting nuclear factor kappa-light-chain-enhancer of activated B cells (NF-κB) activation, reducing inflammatory mediators (NO, PGE2 and TNF-α) and suppressing the release of inflammatory cytokines (IL-1β and IL-6).[55] In an asthma mouse model induced by OVA, *di long* 地龙 alleviated airway hyper-responsiveness, decreased inflammatory mediators (IL-4, IL-5 and IL-13) and downregulated IgE. In addition, it attenuated mucus secretion and infiltration of inflammatory cells in the lungs, while inhibiting the activation of NF-κB signalling.[56] Combined with *wu wei zi* 五味子, it also inhibited infiltration and diffusion of inflammatory cells in a guinea pig asthma model,[57] demonstrating anti-asthmatic effects and potential benefit as a treatment for CVA.

Experimental Studies on *Wu Wei Zi* 五味子

Two species of *wu wei zi* 五味子 are commonly used in CM, *Schisandra chinensis* (Turcz.) Baill. and *Schisandra sphenanthera* Rehd. & Wils. Its main compound groups include lignans (e.g. schisandrin A–C and gomisin), glycosides and organic acid.[7,8]

Antitussive Actions

Wu wei zi 五味子 and its polysaccharides were tested in cough hypersensitivity guinea pig models (both chronic and acute cough).[58,59] Cough frequency and pulmonary inflammation in the cough hyper-sensitivity guinea pigs induced by 14 days of cigarette smoke was significantly reduced by *wu wei zi* 五味子. Pre-treatment also attenuated the increase in infiltration of pulmonary neutrophils and total inflammatory cells, as well as pro-inflammatory cytokines.[59] The authors concluded that the lignans are likely to be the active components including schizandrin, schisantherin A, deoxyschizandrin and γ-schisandrin. In another study, *wu wei zi* 五味子 polysaccharides at 250, 500 and 1000 mg/kg significantly supressed cough compared to codeine. In addition, inflammatory cells in BALF and markers of airway inflammation were attenuated. At 500 mg/kg, cough was suppressed for the whole experiment (five hours), compared to codeine that showed no significant positive effects.[58]

Anti-inflammatory Actions

Wu wei zi 五味子 compounds, such as schisandrin and gomisin, have antiallergy and anti-inflammatory properties by inhibiting kinase activity.[60,61] In terms of inflammation, the effects are likely to occur through inhibition of NF-κB-dependent inflammatory pathways and suppression of MAPK activation.[62] In alveolar epithelial cells and a pulmonary inflammation mouse model, *wu wei zi* 五味子 reduced NO and IL-8, as well as inhibited neutrophils and macrophages, thereby reducing pathological changes in the lungs.[63] *Wu wei zi* 五味子 can also lower airway hyper-responsiveness, IgE and immune cell infiltration in mice with asthma.[64] These effects may be an important benefit for CVA chronic cough because airway remodelling and structural changes are common.[2]

Experimental Studies on *Zi Wan* 紫菀

Aster tataricus L. f. includes bioactive compounds such as saponins (e.g. astersaponins A–H), monoterpene glycosides (e.g. shionosides A–B), flavonoids (e.g. quercetin), triterpines (e.g. shionone) and volatile oils.[8] Reported in materia medica to possess antitussive effects and used to treat cough. Compounds from *zi wan* 紫菀 have anti-oxidant, anti-cancer and antitussive actions.[65–67]

Antitussive Actions

Zi wan 紫菀 was orally administrated to mice and had significant expectorant, antitussive and anti-inflammatory effects. The authors concluded that the main constituents act in a synergistic way and are responsible for the expectorant and antitussive activities potentially by eliminating or alleviating tracheal inflammation (an origin of cough and sputum).[68] The constituent compound shionone has also shown expectorant and antitussive activities in mouse models, as has the volatile oil acetoxy-2-ene(*E*)-4,6-decandiyne.[67,69]

Anti-inflammatory Actions

Aster saponins isolated from *zi wan* 紫菀 were assessed in LPS-stimulated murine macrophages. Saponin B exhibited potent inhibitory activity on NO formation, as well as dose-dependently suppressing nitric oxide synthase (iNOS) and cyclooxygenase-2 (COX-2) protein levels.[70] The anti-inflammatory mechanism acted by attenuating the phosphorylation and degradation of the inhibitor of NF-κB (IκB), in turn blocking NF-κB p65 translocation to the nucleus. In a network pharmacology model of acute lung injury, *zi wan* 紫菀 interacted with four biological processes, and showed potential to inhibit the release of inflammatory cytokines and promote the repair of vascular endothelial.[71] A related herb with similar bioactive compounds, *Aster yomena*, reduced airway hyper-responsiveness in an OVA-sensitised mouse model. *Aster yomena* extract suppressed Th2 responses and enzymes associated with the production of inflammatory mediators, reducing cytokines and eosinophils in BALF and IgE in serum. It also decreases airway hyper-responsiveness and histopathological changes in the lungs.[72]

Experimental Studies on *Ban Xia* 半夏

Ban xia 半夏 (*Pinellia ternata* (Thunb.) Breit.) contains alkaloids, triterpenes, volatile oils and phytosteroles.[7,8] Due to the nature of Chinese herbal medicine, when prescribing *ban xia* 半夏, it is often combined with other herbs such as *chen pi* 陈皮 and *gan cao* 甘草. Therefore, few experiential studies have evaluated crude extracts for antitussive or anti-inflammatory effects. However, one of its bioactive compounds, β-sitosterol, which is also found in a variety of other plants, has been extensively researched. Beta-sitosterol has antioxidant and anti-inflammatory properties, such as reducing eosinophils, intracellular reactive oxygen species (ROS) and inflammatory cytokines. In an OVA-induced asthmatic mouse model, β-sitosterol reduced lung inflammation.[73] Total cells and eosinophils in the BALF markedly decreased after β-sitosterol administration (1mg/kg i.p.). Beta-sitosterol also inhibited IgE, indicating its potential benefit for chronic lung inflammation.

Relevant to GORD, *ban xia* 半夏 has gastric motility and antireflux effects. Gastric emptying after *ban xia* 半夏 herbal combination (*Xiao ban xia tang*) 小半夏汤 was evaluated in mice. The herbs restored metoclopramide-induced propulsion and potentiated methylneostigmine-induced gastric emptying enhancement, therefore regulating gastric motility.[74]

Experimental Studies on *Zi Su Ye* 紫苏叶

The leaf of *Perilla frutescens* (L.) Britt. is commonly used for cough, nasal congestion and common colds, as well as promoting stomach function in CM. Bioactive constituents include volatile oils such as perilla aldehyde, α-pinene, β-pinene, perillanin and other constituents including phenolic acids, essential oils, triterpenes, carotenoids, phytosterols and fatty acids.[8,75]

Antitussive Actions

Zi su ye 紫苏叶 oil improved lung function in an asthma guinea pig model.[76] A constituent compound, luteolin (flavonoid) relaxed histamine-, carbachol- and potassium chloride-induced pre-contractions and inhibited cumulative histamine- and carbachol-induced contractions in guinea pig trachea, demonstrating its relaxant action and potential anti-cough effects.[77]

Anti-inflammatory Actions

In LPS-stimulated lung inflammation in mice, *zi su ye* 紫苏叶 inhibited proinflammatory cytokine (e.g. TNF-α) production in the lung at 100 mg/kg. Phenylpropanoids isolated from *zi su ye* 紫苏叶 were then investigated in lung alveolar epithelial cells. They inhibited IL-6 production at concentrations of 10–100 μM, suggesting they have inhibitory effects against lung inflammation.[78] Other monoterpenoid, alkaloid and flavonoid compounds isolated from *zi su ye* 紫苏叶 show inhibitory effects on proinflammatory cytokines and inflammatory mediators in LPS-stimulated macrophages and mice, indicating broad anti-inflammatory effects.[79,80] Due to its chemical makeup including phenolic acids, flavonoids and carotenoids, *zi su ye* 紫苏叶 also has significant antioxidant capacity.[75]

In CM the leaf is commonly used but the seeds also have therapeutic properties. The seed oil from *Perilla frutescens* protected against reflux oesophagitis in rats. It significantly inhibited gastric secretion, total acidity and oesophagitis index. Combined with *in vitro* results, the authors reported antisecretory (anticholinergic and antihistaminic), antioxidant and lipoxygenase inhibitory activities.[81] *In vitro* and *in vivo* anti-asthmatic effects have been shown in guinea pigs. *Perilla frutescens* seed oil improved lung function by regulating eicosanoid production and suppressing leukotriene generation.[76]

Antiallergic Actions

Zi su ye 紫苏叶 inhibits allergic reactions *in vivo* and *in vitro*.[82] In an OVA-sensitised allergic asthma murine model, Th2 responses, airway inflammation and hyper-reactivity were alleviated.[83] Rosmarinic acid from *zi su ye* 紫苏叶 (1.5 mg/mouse, orally) prevented the increase in eosinophils in BALF in murine airways. It also reduced the expression of IL-4 and IL-5, eotaxin (chemokine) and allergen-specific IgG1 in the lungs of mice, suggesting antiallergic effects for asthma.[84] In another study, *zi su ye* 紫苏叶 and its active compound, rosmarinic acid, ameliorated allergic inflammatory reactions, suggesting an effect on allergic rhinitis and allergic rhinoconjunctivitis.[85]

Other Herbs for Chronic Cough

Several herbs used for specific types of chronic cough were not in the top ten list of all herbs in the RCTs. However they may have important actions relevant to cough suppression and inflammation. For UACS, *bai qian* 白前 was commonly used. *Bai qian* 白前 (*Cynanchum stauntonii* var. *glaucescens*) is traditionally used for cough with phlegm, and its bioactive constituents include triterpene saponins (e.g. glaucosides and glaucogenin), glaucobiose, β-sitosterol and fatty acids.[84] It has various mechanisms attributable to its bioactive compounds such as anti-cancer, anti-inflammatory and antivirus actions.[86] Crude extracts of *bai qian* 白前 showed antitussive and expectorant effects in cough models in mice and anti-asthma benefits in guinea pigs.[87,88] It also showed potent attenuation of acetylcholine- and carbachol-induced contractions in rat trachea, indicating relaxant activities.[89] Cynatratoside B, a steroidal glycoside isolated from *bai qian* 白前 has potent airway smooth muscle relaxant effects.[90] Other compounds, such as β-sitosterol, also have antioxidant and anti-inflammatory properties, as described previously.

Herbs used in GORD-C studies were somewhat different to the other types of herbs. These include *chai hu* 柴胡, *bai shao* 茯苓 and *fu ling* 茯苓, in addition to the cough-specific herbs. *Chai hu* 柴胡 is the root of *Bupleurum chinense* DC. and *Bupleurum scorzonerifolium* Willd. It has over 200 constituent compounds including triterpenoid saponins, polyacetylenes, flavonoids, lignans, essential oils, fatty acids and sterols.[91] *Chai hu* 柴胡 compounds have multiple actions including inhibition of inflammation. GORD-C has an inflammatory component where reflux causes structural and inflammatory airway changes. There are a limited number of relevant studies on *chai hu* 柴胡; however, there are many studies related to its effect on intestinal-inflammation-related digestive diseases. Similar to *chai hu* 柴胡, *fu ling* 茯苓 (*Poria cocos* (Schw.) Wolf) and *bai shao* 茯苓 (*Paeonia lactiflora* Pall.) were commonly identified in clinical studies due to their traditional use to regulate the Liver and tonify the Spleen to reduce dysfunction causing reflux. These herbs have various pharmacological effects, including anti-inflammatory, antioxidative, immune-regulating and anti-cancer properties.[92–94] However, there is limited evidence to suggest they have a direct mechanism to treat reflux-related cough.

Summary of Pharmacological Actions of the Common Herbs

The herbs commonly used in clinical trials for chronic cough have received a significant amount of research attention in experimental models. Crude extracts, including constituent compounds such as polysaccharides and flavonoids, have shown notable antitussive activities.[95] In addition, several herbs with triterpenoid saponins have expectorant actions such as *jie geng's* platycodins and *zi wan's* shion-ones. There are still a limited number of chronic cough models and the majority of included experimental studies focused on surrogate outcomes such as anti-inflammation, antioxidation or immunomodulation. However, chronic non-specific inflammation in the airway is regarded as an important factor in chronic cough.[96] Many antitussive herbs are likely to have antispasmodic or bronchodilator actions, although these effects are yet to be explored in experimental models. The research indicates that herbs have important actions that interact and modulate the key pathophysiological mechanisms associated with chronic cough. Potentially there are additional benefits of the herbs on associated pathogenesis that have not been fully researched in animal models of cough but show promise. These include, but are not limited to, the inflammatory aspects of UACS and CVA, and the digestive aspect of GORD. Furthermore, existing antitussive agents, such as opioids, have side effects. Therefore, the actions of the herbs along with their reported safety may play an important role in reducing severity, exacerbations and progression of chronic cough.

References

1. Chung KF, Pavord ID. (2008) Prevalence, pathogenesis, and causes of chronic cough. *Lancet* **371(9621):** 1364–1374.
2. Niimi A. (2011) Cough and asthma. *Curr Respir Med Rev* **7(1):** 47–54.
3. Morice AH, Jakes AD, Faruqi S, *et al.* (2014) A worldwide survey of chronic cough: A manifestation of enhanced somatosensory response. *Eur Respir J* **44(5):** 1149–1155.
4. Joad JP, Munch PA, Bric JM, *et al.* (2004) Passive smoke effects on cough and airways in young guinea pigs: Role of brainstem substance P. *Am J Respir Crit Care Med* **169(4):** 499–504.
5. Melzack R, Coderre TJ, Katz J, Vaccarino AL. (2001) Central neuroplasticity and pathological pain. *Ann N Y Acad Sci* **933:** 157–174.
6. Prockop DJ, Oh JY. (2012) Mesenchymal stem/stromal cells (MSCs): Role as guardians of inflammation. *Mol Ther* **20(1):** 14–20.
7. Zhou J, Xie G, Yan X. (2011) *Encyclopedia of Traditional Chinese Medicine: Molecular Structures, Pharmacological Activities, Natural Sources and Applications.* Springer, Berlin.

8. Bensky D, Clavey S, Stoger E. (2004) *Chinese Herbal Medicine: Materia Medica*, 3rd ed. Eastland Press, Seattle.

9. Ma CH, Ma ZQ, Fu Q, Ma SP. (2014) Ma Huang Tang ameliorates asthma though modulation of Th1/Th2 cytokines and inhibition of Th17 cells in ovalbumin-sensitized mice. *Chin J Nat Med* **12(5):** 361–366.

10. Fields AM, Kaye AD, Richards TA, *et al.* (2003) Pulmonary vascular responses to ma huang extract. *J Altern Complement Med* **9(5):** 727–733.

11. Poliacek I, Morris KF, Lindsey BG, *et al.* (2011) Blood pressure changes alter tracheobronchial cough: Computational model of the respiratory-cough network and in vivo experiments in anesthetized cats. *J Appl Physiol (1985)* **111(3):** 861–873.

12. Ziment I, Tashkin DP. (2000) Alternative medicine for allergy and asthma. *J Allergy Clin Immunol* **106(4):** 603–614.

13. Zhang Q, Ye M. (2009) Chemical analysis of the Chinese herbal medicine Gan-Cao (licorice). *J Chromatogr A* **1216(11):** 1954–1569.

14. Kamei J, Nakamura R, Ichiki H, Kubo M. (2003) Antitussive principles of Glycyrrhizae radix, a main component of the Kampo preparations Bakumondo-to (Mai-men-dong-tang). *Eur J Pharmacol* **469(1–3):** 159–163.

15. Kamei J, Saitoh A, Asano T, *et al.* (2005) Pharmacokinetic and pharmacodynamic profiles of the antitussive principles of Glycyrrhizae radix (licorice), a main component of the Kampo preparation Bakumondo-to (Mai-men-dong-tang). *Eur J Pharmacol* **507(1–3):** 163–168.

16. Nosalova G, Fleskova D, Jurecek L, *et al.* (2013) Herbal polysaccharides and cough reflex. *Respir Physiol Neurobiol* **187(1):** 47–51.

17. Liu B, Yang J, Wen Q, Li Y. (2008) Isoliquiritigenin, a flavonoid from licorice, relaxes guinea-pig tracheal smooth muscle in vitro and in vivo: Role of cGMP/PKG pathway. *Eur J Pharmacol* **587(1–3):** 257–266.

18. Minamizawa K, Goto H, Shimada Y, *et al.* (2006) Effects of eppika-hangeto, a Kampo formula, and Ephedrae herba against citric acid-induced laryngeal cough in guinea pigs. *J Pharmacol Sci* **101(2):** 118–125.

19. Saha S, Nosal'ova G, Ghosh D, *et al.* (2011) Structural features and in vivo antitussive activity of the water extracted polymer from Glycyrrhiza glabra. *Int J Biol Macromol* **48(4):** 634–638.

20. Anderson DM, Smith WG. (1961) The antitussive activity of glycyrrhetinic acid and its derivatives. *J Pharm Pharmacol* **13:** 396–404.

21. Shakeri F, Ghorani V, Saadat S, *et al.* (2019) The stimulatory effects of medicinal plants on beta2-adrenoceptors of tracheal smooth muscle. *Iran J Allergy Asthma Immunol* **18(1):** 12–26.

22. Obolentseva GV, Litvinenko VI, Ammosov AS, *et al.* (1999) Pharmacological and therapeutic properties of licorice preparations: A review. *Pharm Chem J* **33(8):** 427–434.

23. Ma C, Ma Z, Liao XL, *et al.* (2013) Immunoregulatory effects of glycyrrhizic acid exerts anti-asthmatic effects via modulation of Th1/Th2 cytokines and enhancement of CD4(+)CD25(+)Foxp3+ regulatory T cells in ovalbumin-sensitized mice. *J Ethnopharmacol* **148(3):** 755–762.

24. Yang N, Patil S, Zhuge J, *et al.* (2013) Glycyrrhiza uralensis flavonoids present in anti-asthma formula, ASHMI, inhibit memory Th2 responses in vitro and in vivo. *Phytother Res* **27(9):** 1381–1391.

25. Chu X, Jiang L, Wei M, *et al.* (2013) Attenuation of allergic airway inflammation in a murine model of asthma by Licochalcone A. *Immunopharmacol Immunotoxicol* **35(6):** 653–661.

26. Ram A, Mabalirajan U, Das M, *et al.* (2006) Glycyrrhizin alleviates experimental allergic asthma in mice. *Int Immunopharmacol* **6(9):** 1468–1477.

27. Han S, Sun L, He F, Che H. (2017) Anti-allergic activity of glycyrrhizic acid on IgE-mediated allergic reaction by regulation of allergy-related immune cells. *Sci Rep* **7(1):** 7222.

28. Chen G, Zhu L, Liu Y, *et al.* (2009) Isoliquiritigenin, a flavonoid from licorice, plays a dual role in regulating gastrointestinal motility in vitro and in vivo. *Phytother Res* **23(4):** 498–506.

29. Sadra A, Kweon HS, Huh SO, Cho J. (2017) Gastroprotective and gastric motility benefits of AD-lico/Healthy Gut Glycyrrhiza inflata extract. *Anim Cells Syst (Seoul)* **21(4):** 255–262.

30. Yang Y, Wang S, Bao YR, *et al.* (2017) Anti-ulcer effect and potential mechanism of licoflavone by regulating inflammation mediators and amino acid metabolism. *J Ethnopharmacol* **199:** 175–182.

31. Bolarinwa IF, Orfila C, Morgan MR. (2014) Amygdalin content of seeds, kernels and food products commercially available in the UK. *Food Chem* **152:** 133–139.

32. Miyagoshi M, Amagaya S, Ogihara Y. (1986) Antitussive effects of L-ephedrine, amygdalin, and makyokansekito (Chinese traditional medicine) using a cough model induced by sulfur dioxide gas in mice. *Planta Med* **(4):** 275–278.

33. Lin YC, Chang CW, Wu CR. (2016) Antitussive, anti-pyretic and toxicological evaluation of Ma-Xing-Gan-Shi-Tang in rodents. *BMC Complement Altern Med* **16(1):** 456.

34. Vardi N, Parlakpinar H, Ates B, *et al.* (2013) The protective effects of Prunus armeniaca L. (apricot) against methotrexate-induced oxidative damage and apoptosis in rat kidney. *J Physiol Biochem* **69(3):** 371–381.

35. Lee HH, Ahn JH, Kwon AR, *et al.* (2014) Chemical composition and antimicrobial activity of the essential oil of apricot seed. *Phytother Res* **28(12):** 1867–1872.

36. Yigit D, Yigit N, Mavi A. (2009) Antioxidant and antimicrobial activities of bitter and sweet apricot (Prunus armeniaca L.) kernels. *Braz J Med Biol Res* **42(4):** 346–352.

37. Jung KH, Choi HL, Park S, *et al.* (2014) The effects of the standardized herbal formula PM014 on pulmonary inflammation and airway responsiveness in a murine model of cockroach allergen-induced asthma. *J Ethnopharmacol* **155(1):** 113–122.

38. He Y, Lou X, Jin Z, *et al.* (2018) Mahuang decoction mitigates airway inflammation and regulates IL-21/STAT3 signaling pathway in rat asthma model. *J Ethnopharmacol* **224:** 373–380.

39. Lee H, Kim Y, Kim HJ, *et al.* (2012) Herbal formula, PM014, attenuates lung inflammation in a murine model of chronic obstructive pulmonary disease. *Evid Based Complement Alternat Med* **2012:** 769830.

40. Do JS, Hwang JK, Seo HJ, *et al.* (2006) Antiasthmatic activity and selective inhibition of type 2 helper T cell response by aqueous extract of semen armeniacae amarum. *Immunopharmacol Immunotoxicol* **28(2):** 213–225.

41. Jiang H, Yang S, Chen H. (2017) Screening of effective parts of cicada slough for relieving cough, phlegm and asthma. *Mod Chin Med* **19(1):** 56–59.

42. Xu S, Zhang M, Wang Y. (2007) Pharmacological study on antitussive, expectorant and antiasthmatic effects of cicada slough. *Chinese Pharmacological* S377–S382.

43. Kim M, Kim H, Ryu J, *et al.* (2014) Anti-inflammatory effects of Cryptotympana atrata Fabricius slough shed on contact dermatitis induced by dinitrofluorobenzene in mice. *Pharmacogn Mag* **10(Suppl 2):** S377–S382.

44. Zhang L, Wang Y, Yang D, *et al.* (2015) Platycodon grandiflorus: An ethnopharmacological, phytochemical and pharmacological review. *J Ethnopharmacol* **164:** 147–161.

45. Sun RR, Zhang MY, Chen Q. (2010) Platycodin capsules inflammatory cough asthma research. *Pharmacology and Clinics of Chinese Materia Medica* **26:** 27–29.

46. Shin CY, Lee WJ, Lee EB, *et al.* (2002) Platycodin D and D3 increase airway mucin release in vivo and in vitro in rats and hamsters. *Planta Med* **68(3):** 221–225.

47. Ryu J, Lee HJ, Park SH, *et al.* (2014) Effects of the root of Platycodon grandiflorum on airway mucin hypersecretion in vivo and platycodin D(3) and deapi-platycodin on production and secretion of airway mucin in vitro. *Phytomedicine* **21(4):** 529–533.

48. Park YJ, Bang IJ, Jung MH, *et al.* (2019) Effects of beta-sitosterol from corn silk on TGF-beta1-induced epithelial-mesenchymal transition in lung alveolar epithelial cells. *J Agric Food Chem* **67(35):** 9789–9795.

49. Chunhua M, Long H, Zhu W, *et al.* (2017) Betulin inhibited cigarette smoke-induced COPD in mice. *Biomed Pharmacother* **85:** 679–686.

50. Gao W, Guo Y, Yang H. (2017) Platycodin D protects against cigarette smoke-induced lung inflammation in mice. *Int Immunopharmacol* **47:** 53–58.

51. Lee JH, Choi YH, Kang HS, Choi BT. (2004) An aqueous extract of Platycodi radix inhibits LPS-induced NF-kappaB nuclear translocation in human cultured airway epithelial cells. *Int J Mol Med* **13(6):** 843–847.

52. Choi JH, Hwang YP, Lee HS, Jeong HG. (2009) Inhibitory effect of Platycodi Radix on ovalbumin-induced airway inflammation in a murine model of asthma. *Food Chem Toxicol* **47(6):** 1272–1279.

53. Chu X, Xu Z, Wu D, *et al.* (2007) In vitro and in vivo evaluation of the anti-asthmatic activities of fractions from Pheretima. *J Ethnopharmacol* **111(3):** 490–495.

54. Barnes PJ. (2006) Drugs for asthma. *Br J Pharmacol* **147(Suppl 1):** S297–S303.

55. Huang C, Li W, Zhang Q, *et al.* (2018) Anti-inflammatory activities of Guang-Pheretima extract in lipopolysaccharide-stimulated RAW 264.7 murine macrophages. *BMC Complement Altern Med* **18(1):** 46.

56. Huang CQ, Li W, Wu B, *et al.* (2016) Pheretima aspergillum decoction suppresses inflammation and relieves asthma in a mouse model of bronchial asthma by NF-kappaB inhibition. *J Ethnopharmacol* **189:** 22–30.

57. Li XH, Tu XY, Zhang DX, *et al.* (2009) Effects of wuwei dilong decoction on inflammatory cells and cytokines in asthma model guinea pigs. *J Tradit Chin Med* **29(3):** 220–223.

58. Zhong S, Liu XD, Nie YC, *et al.* (2016) Antitussive activity of the Schisandra chinensis fruit polysaccharide (SCFP-1) in guinea pigs models. *J Ethnopharmacol* **194:** 378–385.

59. Zhong S, Nie YC, Gan ZY, *et al.* (2015) Effects of Schisandra chinensis extracts on cough and pulmonary inflammation in a cough hypersensitivity guinea pig model induced by cigarette smoke exposure. *J Ethnopharmacol* **165:** 73–82.

60. Guo LY, Hung TM, Bae KH, *et al.* (2008) Anti-inflammatory effects of schisandrin isolated from the fruit of Schisandra chinensis Baill. *Eur J Pharmacol* **591(1–3):** 293–299.

61. Oh SY, Kim YH, Bae DS, *et al.* (2010) Anti-inflammatory effects of gomisin N, gomisin J, and schisandrin C isolated from the fruit of Schisandra chinensis. *Biosci Biotechnol Biochem* **74(2):** 285–291.

62. Kang YS, Han MH, Hong SH, *et al.* (2014) Anti-inflammatory effects of Schisandra chinensis (Turcz.) Baill fruit through the inactivation of nuclear factor-kappaB and mitogen-activated protein kinases signaling pathways in lipopolysaccharide-stimulated murine macrophages. *J Cancer Prev* **19(4):** 279–287.

63. Bae H, Kim R, Kim Y, *et al.* (2012) Effects of Schisandra chinensis Baillon (Schizandraceae) on lipopolysaccharide induced lung inflammation in mice. *J Ethnopharmacol* **142(1):** 41–47.

64. Kim H, Ahn YT, Kim YS, *et al.* (2014) Antiasthmatic effects of Schizandrae fructus extract in mice with asthma. *Pharmacogn Mag* **10(Suppl 1):** S80–S85.

65. Ng TB, Liu F, Lu Y, *et al.* (2003) Antioxidant activity of compounds from the medicinal herb Aster tataricus. *Comp Biochem Physiol C Toxicol Pharmacol* **136(2):** 109–115.

66. Du L, Mei HF, Yin X, Xing YQ. (2014) Delayed growth of glioma by a polysaccharide from Aster tataricus involve upregulation of Bax/Bcl-2 ratio, activation of caspase-3/8/9, and downregulation of the Akt. *Tumour Biol* **35(3):** 1819–1825.

67. Yang B, Xiao YQ, Liang RX, *et al.* (2008) [Studies on expectorant compounds in volatile oil from root and rhizome of Aster tataricus]. *Zhongguo Zhong Yao Za Zhi* **33(3):** 281–283.

68. Yu P, Cheng S, Xiang J, *et al.* (2015) Expectorant, antitussive, anti-inflammatory activities and compositional analysis of Aster tataricus. *J Ethnopharmacol* **164:** 328–333.

69. Lu YH, Dai Y, Wang ZT, Xu LS. (1999) Expectorant and antitussive effects of Aster tataricus and its active constituents. *Chinese Traditional and Herbal Drugs* **30:** 360–362.

70. Su XD, Jang HJ, Wang CY, *et al.* (2019) Anti-inflammatory potential of saponins from Aster tataricus via NF-kappaB/MAPK activation. *J Nat Prod* **82(5):** 1139–1148.

71. Chen Y, Dong J, Liu J, *et al.* (2019) Network pharmacology-based investigation of protective mechanism of Aster tataricus on lipopolysaccharide-induced acute lung injury. *Int J Mol Sci* **20(3):** 543.

72. Sim JH, Lee HS, Lee S, *et al.* (2014) Anti-asthmatic activities of an ethanol extract of Aster yomena in an ovalbumin-induced murine asthma model. *J Med Food* **17(5):** 606–611.

73. Yuk JE, Woo JS, Yun CY, *et al.* (2007) Effects of lactose-beta-sitosterol and beta-sitosterol on ovalbumin-induced lung inflammation in actively sensitized mice. *Int Immunopharmacol* **7(12):** 1517–1527.

74. Chen D, Wu CF, Huang L, Ning Z. (2002) Effect of the aqueous extract of xiao-ban-xia-tang on gastric emptying in mice. *Am J Chin Med.* **30(2–3):** 207–214.

75. Ahmed HM. (2018) Ethnomedicinal, phytochemical and pharmacological investigations of Perilla frutescens (L.) Britt. *Molecules* **24(1):** 102.

76. Deng YM, Xie QM, Zhang SJ, *et al.* (2007) Anti-asthmatic effects of Perilla seed oil in the guinea pig in vitro and in vivo. *Planta Med* **73(1):** 53–58.

77. Ko WC, Shih CM, Leu IJ, *et al.* (2005) Mechanisms of relaxant action of luteolin in isolated guinea pig trachea. *Planta Med* **71(5):** 406–411.

78. Lim HJ, Woo KW, Lee KR, *et al.* (2014) Inhibition of Proinflammatory cytokine generation in lung inflammation by the leaves of Perilla frutescens and its constituents. *Biomol Ther (Seoul).* **22(1):** 62–67.

79. Ueda H, Yamazaki C, Yamazaki M. (2002) Luteolin as an anti-inflammatory and anti-allergic constituent of Perilla frutescens. *Biol Pharm Bull* **25(9):** 1197–1202.

80. Wang XF, Li H, Jiang K, *et al.* (2018) Anti-inflammatory constituents from Perilla frutescens on lipopolysaccharide-stimulated RAW264.7 cells. *Fitoterapia* **130:** 61–65.

81. Arya E, Saha S, Saraf SA, Kaithwas G. (2013) Effect of Perilla frutescens fixed oil on experimental esophagitis in albino Wistar rats. *Biomed Res Int* **2013:** 981372.

82. Yu H, Qiu JF, Ma LJ, *et al.* (2017) Phytochemical and phytopharmacological review of Perilla frutescens L. (Labiatae), a traditional edible-medicinal herb in China. *Food Chem Toxicol* **108(Pt B):** 375–391.

83. Chen ML, Wu CH, Hung LS, Lin BF. (2015) Ethanol extract of Perilla frutescens suppresses allergen-specific Th2 Responses and alleviates airway inflammation and hyperreactivity in ovalbumin-sensitized murine model of asthma. *Evid Based Complement Alternat Med* **2015:** 324265.

84. Sanbongi C, Takano H, Osakabe N, *et al.* (2004) Rosmarinic acid in perilla extract inhibits allergic inflammation induced by mite allergen, in a mouse model. *Clin Exp Allergy* **34(6):** 971–977.

85. Oh HA, Park CS, Ahn HJ, *et al.* (2011) Effect of Perilla frutescens var. acuta Kudo and rosmarinic acid on allergic inflammatory reactions. *Exp Biol Med (Maywood)* **236(1):** 99–106.

86. Han L, Zhou X, Yang M, *et al.* (2018) Ethnobotany, phytochemistry and pharmacological effects of plants in genus Cynanchum Linn. (Asclepiadaceae). *Molecules* **23(5):** 1194.

87. Liang A, Xue B, Yang Q, *et al.* (1996) [Antitussive, expectorant and anti-inflammatory effects of rhizoma Cynanchi stauntonii]. *Zhongguo Zhong Yao Za Zhi* **21(3):** 173–175, 91–92.

88. Liang A, Xue B, Yang Q, Li Z. (1995) [Antitussive, expectorant and anti-asthmatic effects of Cynanchum glaucescens (Decne.) Hand. -Mazz]. *Zhongguo Zhong Yao Za Zhi* **20(3):** 176–178, inside front cover.

89. Yue GG, Chan BC, Kwok HF, *et al.* (2012) Screening for anti-inflammatory and bronchorelaxant activities of 12 commonly used Chinese herbal medicines. *Phytother Res* **26(6):** 915–925.

90. Yue GG, Chan KM, To MH, *et al.* (2014) Potent airway smooth muscle relaxant effect of cynatratoside B, a steroidal glycoside isolated from Cynanchum stauntonii. *J Nat Prod* **77(4):** 1074–1077.

91. Yang F, Dong X, Yin X, *et al.* (2017) Radix bupleuri: A review of traditional uses, botany, phytochemistry, pharmacology, and toxicology. *Biomed Res Int* **2017:** 7597596.

92. Rios JL. (2011) Chemical constituents and pharmacological properties of Poria cocos. *Planta Med* **77(7):** 681–691.

93. Parker S, May B, Zhang C, *et al.* (2016) A pharmacological review of bioactive constituents of Paeonia lactiflora Pallas and Paeonia veitchii Lynch. *Phytother Res* **30(9):** 1445–1473.

94. He DY, Dai SM. (2011) Anti-inflammatory and immunomodulatory effects of Paeonia lactiflora Pall., a traditional chinese herbal medicine. *Front Pharmacol* **2:** 10.

95. Saraswathy GR, Sathiya R, Anbu J, Maheswari E. (2004) Antitussive medicinal herbs: An update review. *Int J Pharm Sci Drug Res* **6(1):** 12–19.

96. Birring SS. (2011) New concepts in the management of chronic cough. *Pulm Pharmacol Ther* **24(3):** 334–338.

7

Clinical Evidence for Acupuncture and Related Therapies

OVERVIEW

Clinical evidence for acupuncture and related therapies for chronic cough are assessed in this chapter. Five randomised controlled trials were included. Acupuncture was evaluated in three studies, ear acupressure in one study and acupuncture combined with herbal medicine in one study. All of the studies assessed cough variant asthma; there were no clinical trials that assessed upper airway cough syndrome or gastro-oesophageal reflux disease-related cough.

Introduction

Acupuncture is part of a family of techniques which stimulate acupuncture points to correct imbalances of energy and restore health to the body. Acupuncture involves the insertion of acupuncture needles into acupuncture points. Acupuncture is commonly used in clinical practice for respiratory conditions including chronic cough; however, there are only a small number of clinical trials that have assessed its benefits on cough variant asthma (CVA).

Previous Systematic Reviews

The database search did not find any previous systematic reviews evaluating acupuncture or related therapies for chronic cough.

Identification of Clinical Studies

A comprehensive search identified 15,142 citations. After duplicate removal, 4,898 citations were screened and 1,247 underwent full-text review. After exclusions, five randomised controlled trials (RCTs; 346 participants) were included (A1–A5). Non-randomised controlled trials and non-controlled studies were not identified in the search (Fig. 7.1). All studies were conducted in China and published in Chinese.

Characteristics of Clinical Studies

All studies evaluated the effect of acupuncture (A1–A3), ear acupressure (A4), or acupuncture combined with herbal medicine (A5) on CVA. Pharmacotherapies were the comparator in two studies and three studies that administered acupuncture or acupressure alongside pharmacotherapies compared to the same pharmacotherapies alone. The participants' ages ranged from 18 to 62 years and 56.4% were male. Chinese medicine syndrome differentiation was not used in the studies.

The clinical trial published by You *et al.* (2016) compared acupuncture plus cetirizine (a second-generation antihistamine) and montelukast (a leukotriene receptor antagonist), to cetirizine and montelukast alone. Acupuncture was given daily for 45 days at BL12 *Fengmen* 风门, GV14 *Dazhui* 大椎, BL13 *Feishu* 肺俞, BL20 *Pishu* 脾俞 and BL23 *Shenshu* 肾俞 (A1).

Zhang *et al.* (2017) compared acupuncture plus fluticasone and salmeterol (an inhaled corticosteroid and long-acting [β]2 adrenergic receptor agonist), terbutaline (a short-acting β2 adrenergic receptor agonist) and montelukast, to the same drugs alone. Acupuncture was given every second day for four weeks at BL13 *Feishu* 肺俞, EX-B1 *Dingchuan* 定喘, BL43 *Gaohuang* 膏肓, LU7 *Lieque* 列缺, ST36 *Zusanli* 足三里 and ST40 *Fenglong* 丰隆 (A2).

Zhang Yan *et al.* (2017) compared acupuncture to budesonide (an inhaled corticosteroid) and montelukast. Acupuncture points included LU10 *Yuji* 鱼际, LU5 *Chize* 尺泽, LU7 *Lieque* 列缺, ST36

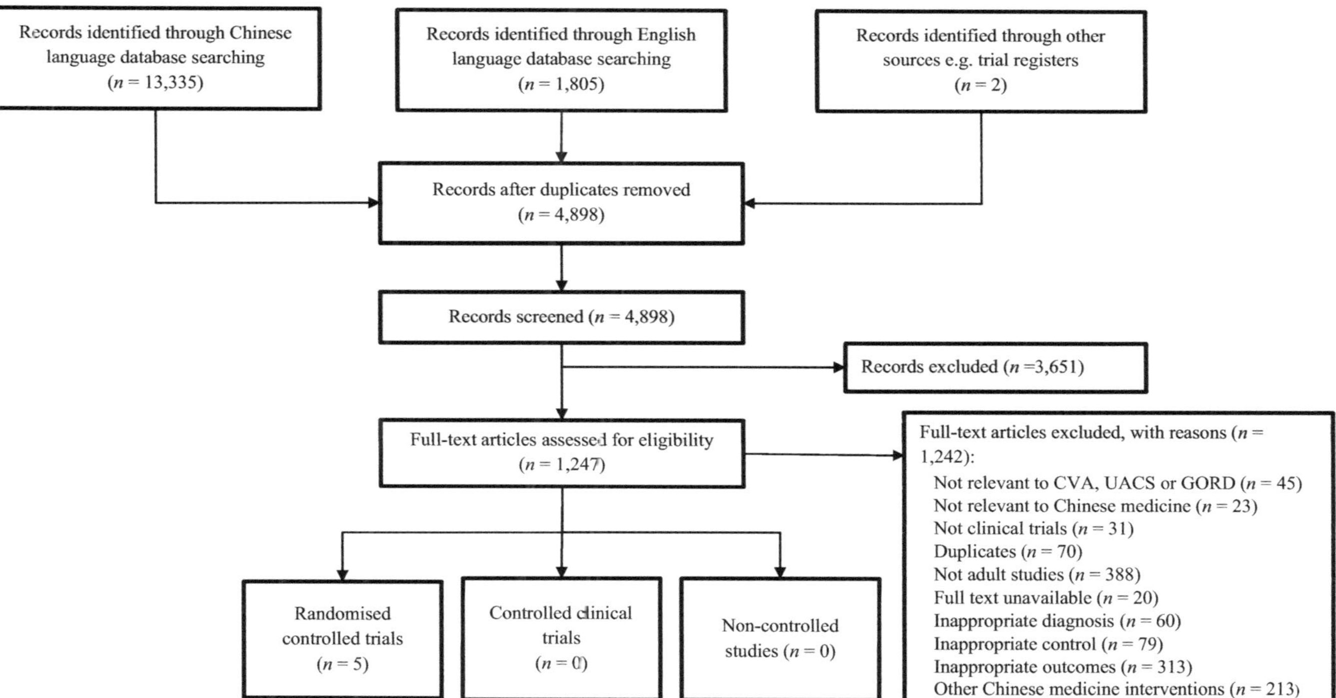

Fig. 7.1. Flowchart of study selection process: Acupuncture and related therapies.

Abbreviations: CVA, cough variant asthma; GORD, gastro-oesophageal reflux disease; UACS, upper airway cough syndrome.

Zusanli 足三里, ST40 *Fenglong* 丰隆, BL13 *Feishu* 肺俞 and BL20 *Pishu* 脾俞, administered every second day for four weeks (A3).

Liu *et al.* (2017) assessed the effect of ear acupressure combined with fluticasone and salmeterol, compared to fluticasone and salmeterol alone. Ear acupressure points included CO14 *Lung* 肺, TF4 *Shenmen* 神门, TG3 *Throat* 咽喉, CO16 *Trachea* 气管, and *Asthma point* 平喘点. Participants were asked to pressure the points four times a day for three to five minutes each time for four weeks (A4).

He *et al.* (2017) used acupuncture combined with the herbal formula *Shu feng jie jing tang* 疏风解痉汤, compared to montelukast for three weeks (A5). Acupuncture included *Jia ji* 夹脊穴 points every second day and herbs included: *Ma huang* 麻黄, *su ye* 苏叶, *xing ren* 杏仁, *fang feng* 防风, *qian hu* 前胡, *zhi ke* 枳壳, *jie geng* 桔梗, *chan tui* 蝉蜕, *wu wei zi* 五味子, *zi wan* 紫菀, *bai bu* 百部, *tao ren* 桃仁, *ju luo* 橘络, *bai shao* 白芍 and *gan cao* 甘草.

All the studies used different methodologies and different acupuncture points, although BL13 *Feishu* 肺俞 was the most common point used in multiple studies. Treatment duration ranged from three weeks to six weeks and long-term results could not be evaluated.

Risk of Bias

Four RCTs used a random number table to generate the allocation sequence, and one did not describe sequence generation (A5). The method of allocation concealment was not described in any of the studies. Blinding of participants and personnel, and outcome assessors was at 'high' risk of bias because the studies were not blind. Data were complete and there was no missing data or drop-outs in the studies, except for one that did not mention relevant information to make a judgment and was rated at 'unclear' risk of bias (A4). Selective outcome reporting was assessed as 'unclear' risk of bias because study protocols were not available.

Outcomes

Effective Rate

All studies evaluated effective rate. Participants in the studies were grouped into one of two groups based on the effectiveness of the treatment, that is, effective or ineffective. The treatment was considered effective if the participant experienced a marked improvement whereby cough was significantly relieved and other objective indicators were noticeably improved, or there was symptom control, where cough returned to the level before the symptoms presented. Treatment was ineffective if the participants did not have a markedly improved effect, or there was no significant improvement. The classification of effective rate was based on clinical judgment, but the outcomes were not validated measures.

Two integrative medicine studies (acupuncture plus pharmacotherapy) were merged in meta-analysis, and results showed that acupuncture plus pharmacotherapy was superior to pharmacotherapy alone (risk ratio [RR]: 1.45 [1.12, 1.88], I^2 = 0%) (A1–A2). The study comparing acupuncture to budesonide and montelukast also showed a positive effect in favour of acupuncture (RR: 1.67 [1.15, 2.42]) (A3). Ear acupressure plus pharmacotherapy was not superior to pharmacotherapy alone (RR: 1.16 [0.78, 1.73]) (A4). Neither was acupuncture combined with herbal medicine, compared to montelukast (RR: 1.31 [0.69, 2.49]) (A5).

Lung Function

Lung function was evaluated after four weeks of acupuncture treatment (A3). Forced expiratory volume in one second (FEV_1), forced vital capacity (FVC) and peak expiratory flow (PEF) significantly improved in the acupuncture group compared to those in the budesonide and montelukast group (mean difference [MD]: 0.76 litres [0.69, 0.83]), (MD: 0.83 litres [0.75, 0.91]) and (MD: 10.84% [8.72, 12.96]), respectively.

Ear acupuncture plus fluticasone and salmeterol was not superior to drugs alone in terms of FEV_1 or PEF after four weeks of treatment

(MD: 2.92% [–6.08, 11.92]) and (MD: 4.98% [–1.55, 11.51]), respectively (A4). Acupuncture combined with herbal medicine was superior to montelukast in terms of FEV_1 (MD: 1.49 litres [1.42, 1.56]), FVC (MD: 0.49 litres [0.39, 0.59]) and PEF (MD: 1.96 litres/second [1.31, 2.61]) (A5).

Cough Symptom Score

One study measured the cough symptom score, a questionnaire that rates the severity of cough from zero to 12, where a lower score indicates less severe cough. After ear acupressure plus fluticasone and salmeterol, the cough symptom score was reduced compared to fluticasone and salmeterol alone (MD: –0.37 [–0.56, –0.18]) (A4).

Eosinophils

Two studies evaluated blood eosinophils, an indicator of inflammation. Acupuncture plus cetirizine and montelukast reduced eosinophil numbers compared to cetirizine and montelukast alone (MD: $–0.32 \times 10^9$/litres [–0.43, –0.21]) (A1). Acupuncture plus herbal medicine also reduced eosinophil numbers compared to montelukast (MD: $–0.17 \times 10^9$/litres [–0.24, –0.10]) (A5).

Safety

One study (A3) reported adverse events. In the acupuncture group there were two reports of gastrointestinal upset. In the control group of budesonide and montelukast there were six cases of gastrointestinal upset, ten cases of blood, liver and kidney abnormalities, and two cases of allergic reaction. However, the severity of adverse events was not reported in either group.

Summary of Acupuncture and Related Therapies Clinical Evidence

Five RCTs of acupuncture, ear acupressure or acupuncture plus herbal medicine for CVA were identified and included in the analysis.

Acupuncture points included those that tonify the Lung, Spleen and Kidney, clear damp and benefit the Lung. BL13 *Feishu* 肺俞 was used in three of the studies and appears to be an important point for the treatment of CVA-type chronic cough. Other common points were LU7 *Lieque* 列缺, ST36 *Zusanli* 足三里 and ST40 *Fenglong* 丰隆 to regulate *qi*, transform phlegm/dampness and stop cough. Ear acupressure points were related to regions of the Lung and Throat. Three to four weeks of treatment with acupuncture, but not ear acupressure, appear to be sufficient to show a trend towards improvement in cough symptoms, lung function and eosinophil counts. However, the studies were small in terms of the number of participants and a clear understanding of acupuncture's effect on CVA cannot be drawn from these studies; yet the results are encouraging.

References for Included Acupuncture Therapies Clinical Studies

Study No.	Reference
A1	尤传静, 吴强, 王光铭. (2016) 针刺配合电磁波疗法治疗咳嗽变异性哮喘 21 例临床研究. 实用中西医结合临床 **16(8):** 12–14.
A2	张丽霞, 李雪青, 石志敏. (2017) 针药结合治疗咳嗽变异性哮喘的临床研究. 针灸临床杂志 **33(1):** 15–17.
A3	张妍, 张磊, 李艳, 朱晓婷, 刘霞, 潘玲玲. (2017) 补土肃肺针法治疗咳嗽变异性哮喘的临床观察. 针灸临床杂志 **33(4):** 6–9.
A4	刘琪, 朱文武. (2017) 耳穴贴压联合沙美特罗丙酸氟替卡松治疗咳嗽变异性哮喘临床研究. 亚太传统医药 **13(10):** 111–112.
A5	何萍萍, 张芙蓉, 杨睿. (2017) 针药并用治疗咳嗽变异性哮喘疗效观察. 上海针灸杂志 **36(11):** 1311–1314.

8

Summary and Conclusions

OVERVIEW

This chapter summarises the main findings of the previous chapters including those from the classical literature, clinical trial evidence and experimental evidence. Chinese medicine therapies, including herbal medicine and acupuncture, are discussed regarding the clinical management of chronic cough. Limitations of the available evidence are reported, and future directions identified for clinical and experimental research. Chinese medicine therapies are commonly used to treat chronic cough, and evidence from historical literature shows that Chinese medicine has been used for thousands of years. Findings from modern clinical trials indicate Chinese medicine is potentially effective and safe for people with chronic cough.

Introduction

Chinese medicine (CM) therapies are increasingly used to treat chronic cough and many clinical studies have been conducted. The three most common types of chronic cough are cough variant asthma (CVA), upper airway cough syndrome (UACS), and gastro-oesophageal reflux disease-related cough (GORD-C), accounting for approximately 90% of cases. These three chronic cough subtypes are the focus of this book.

Current conventional management of chronic cough mainly aims to relieve symptoms. Cough variant asthma treatment is similar to typical asthma due to relatively similar mechanism of disease. First-line treatments include inhaled bronchodilators combined with inhaled corticosteroids (ICS), as well as avoiding cough-inducing triggers, although some patients have side effects from treatment.[1] Treatments for UACS focus on rhinosinusitis management including decongestants, antihistamines, anticholinergics and topical nasal corticosteroids.[2] Treatments for GORD should firstly include diet modification and lifestyle changes, and in patients with chronic cough, heartburn and regurgitation, proton pump inhibitors (PPIs), H2-receptor antagonists, alginate and/or antacid therapies are recommended. However, PPIs do not reduce cough in 30–50% of patients, and are not recommended in people with chronic cough, without heartburn or regurgitation.[3] Chinese medicine treatments may therefore be of value.

This book includes a 'whole-evidence' analysis of CM for the treatment of chronic cough. Clinical guidelines and textbooks (Chapter 2) have recommended a broad range of CM treatments for chronic cough, including oral Chinese herbal medicine (CHM), acupuncture and other CM therapies. Review of the classical literature identified a range of CHMs, acupuncture and other CM therapies which have been used for the management of chronic cough (Chapter 3). Findings from clinical studies revealed promising benefits of oral CHM for chronic cough (Chapter 5). There were only a small number of studies that assessed acupuncture and related therapies, and more research is needed to verify the benefits of these therapies (Chapter 7).

Chinese Medicine Syndrome Differentiation

Current clinical guidelines categorise chronic cough into six syndromes according to the presenting signs and symptoms, including the following:

- Severe wind attacking the Lungs;
- Phlegm-dampness obstructing the Lungs;
- Phlegm congealing in the throat;
- Stomach *qi* ascending upwards;
- Liver fire attacking the Lungs;
- Deficiency of Lung *yin.*

For each syndrome, a single formula or a combined formula is suggested as a guide for clinical practice (Chapter 2). Consistent with contemporary CM literature's understanding of chronic cough, the classical CM literature (Chapter 3) also included citations that detailed the dysfunction of different *zang fu* organs leading to chronic cough. Fire, heat and dryness were the most frequently mentioned pathogens in the included citations that caused disordered diffusion of Lung *qi* manifesting as chronic cough.

In randomised controlled trials (RCTs) of CVA and UACS, about 50% included a CM syndrome classification. In studies that described CM syndromes, the most common syndromes included severe wind attacking the Lungs and wind-phlegm obstructing the Lungs. The former is consistent with that mentioned in the clinical practice guidelines (Chapter 2). In RCTs of GORD-C, CM syndrome classification was used in two studies and included Liver depression, Spleen deficiency and Stomach *qi* ascending. In the five acupuncture and related therapy studies, CM syndrome differentiation was not used. Syndrome differentiation could not be used as a classifying factor to pool studies for analysis if a particular syndrome was more or less effective in producing a positive effect in the clinical studies. This was due to the large number of different syndromes.

Chinese Herbal Medicine

This section summarises the evidence from Chapter 2, Chapter 3 and Chapter 5. Overall, the CHMs commonly used for chronic cough are consistent between classical literature, contemporary clinical guidelines and clinical trials (Table 8.1). Chinese herbal medicine for chronic cough was evaluated in 193 RCTs, seven non-randomised controlled clinical trials (CCTs) and 12 non-controlled studies. Among them, 180 studies were related to CVA, 14 studies related to UACS and 18 studies related to GORD-C. All the studies were conducted in China.

A considerable number of instruments assessed cough severity. The instruments with sufficient data suitable for pooling were effective

Table 8.1.   Summary of Chinese Herbal Medicine Formulas

Formula Name	Included in Clinical Guidelines and Textbooks (Chapter 2)	Included in Classical Literature (Chapter 3) (No. of Citations)	Included in Clinical Studies (Chapter 5)								
			RCTs (No. of Studies)			CCTs (No. of Studies)			NCS (No. of Studies)		
			CVA	UACS	GORD-C	CVA	UACS	GORD-C	CVA	UACS	GORD-C
Su huang zhi ke fang 苏黄止咳方	Yes	0	24	0	0	0	0	0	0	0	0
Er chen tang 二陈汤 combined with *San zi yang qin tang* 三子养亲汤	Yes	0	0	0	0	0	0	0	0	0	0
Qing yan li qiao tang 清咽利窍汤	Yes	0	0	0	0	0	0	0	0	0	0
Xuan fu dai zhe tang 旋覆代赭汤 combined with *Ban xia xie xin tang* 半夏泻心汤	Yes	0	1	0	0	0	0	0	0	0	0
Dai ge san 黛蛤散 combined with *Huang qin xie bai san* 黄芩泻白散	Yes	0	0	0	0	0	0	0	0	0	0

Sha shen mai dong tang 沙参麦冬汤	Yes	0	0	0	0	0	0	0	0	0	0
E jiao san 阿胶散	No	9	0	0	0	0	0	0	0	0	0
Bei mu tang 贝母汤	No	5	0	0	0	0	0	0	0	0	0
Bu fei tang 补肺汤	No	5	0	0	0	0	0	0	0	0	0
Ga jie wan 蛤蚧丸	No	5	0	0	0	0	0	0	0	0	0
Zi wan san 紫菀散	No	5	0	0	0	0	0	0	0	0	0
Bei mu wan 贝母丸	No	3	0	0	0	0	0	0	0	0	0
He zi yin 诃子饮	No	3	0	0	0	0	0	0	0	0	0
Jin su wan 金粟丸	No	3	0	0	0	0	0	0	0	0	0
Jiu sou wan zi 久嗽丸子	No	3	0	0	0	0	0	0	0	0	0
Ren shen kuan hua gao 人参款花膏	No	3	0	0	0	0	0	0	0	0	0
Zhi ke tang 枳壳汤	No	3	0	0	0	0	0	0	0	0	0
Zhou fei wan 皱肺丸	No	3	0	0	0	0	0	0	0	0	0
Zi wan wan 紫菀丸	No	3	0	0	0	0	0	0	0	0	0
Zhi sou san 止嗽散	No	0	9	1	0	1	0	0	1	0	0
Xiao qing long tang 小青龙汤	No	0	6	0	0	0	0	0	0	0	0
Wen dan tang 温胆汤	No	0	4	0	0	0	0	0	0	0	0

The total number of studies in each section included 355 classical literature citations, 193 RCTs, seven CCTs and 12 non-controlled studies. Abbreviations: CCTs, controlled clinical trials; CVA, cough variant asthma; GORD-C, gastro-oesophageal reflux disease-related cough; NCS, non-controlled studies; RCTs, randomised controlled trials; UACS, upper airway cough syndrome.

rate, lung function forced expiratory volume in one second (FEV$_1$), peak expiratory flow (PEF), forced vital capacity (FVC), blood eosinophil count (EOS) and cough symptom score. Other outcomes such as the Leicester cough questionnaire (LCQ), visual analogue scales (VAS), eosinophil cationic protein (ECP), exhaled nitric oxide (FeNO) and cough reflex sensitivity were not commonly used.

Compared to placebo, CHM reduced cough symptom score and VAS, and improved total effective rate. Compared to pharmacotherapy, CHM reduced cough symptom score, VAS and ECP, and improved LCQ scores, FEV$_1$ and total effective rate; however, heterogeneity was 'high'. Chinese herbal medicine reduced FeNO, compared to pharmacotherapies, and heterogeneity was 'low'.

Compared to pharmacotherapy, CHM plus pharmacotherapy improved LCQ scores and reduced cough symptom scores, although heterogeneity was 'high'. The integrative medicine also improved total effective rate, FEV$_1$, FVC (litres), PEF (percent), and PEF (litres/second), but heterogeneity remained 'high'. However, ECP and VAS were reduced, and heterogeneity was 'low'. Moreover, CHM alone, or given as integrative medicine, did not significantly change eosinophil counts.

Risk of bias

Although some of the results were positive, the studies were not free from bias, and heterogeneity was substantial in most of the meta-analysis results. Safety outcomes, such as adverse events, were reported in 32.6% of studies. For CVA studies, 39.2% were at 'low' risk of bias for sequence generation and 59.0% were at 'unclear' risk of bias for sequence generation. Furthermore, 97.6% were assessed as 'unclear' risk of bias for allocation concealment, and 99.4% at 'high' risk of bias for blinding of participants and personnel. All studies were at 'high' risk of bias for blinding of outcome assessors and 98.8% at 'unclear' risk of bias for selective reporting.

For UACS studies, 81.8% were at 'unclear' risk of bias for sequence generation and 100% were at 'unclear' risk of bias for allocation concealment and selective outcome reporting. Furthermore,

81.8% were at 'high' risk of bias for blinding of participants and blinding of personnel and 100% were at 'high' risk of bias for blinding of outcome assessors. For GORD-C studies, 62.5% were assessed as 'unclear' risk of bias for sequence generation and 93.8% were at 'unclear' risk of bias for allocation concealment and selective outcome reporting. All of the studies were at 'high' risk of bias for blinding of participants, personnel and outcome assessors. In summary, the methodological quality was 'low' to 'moderate', and results should be interpreted with caution because none of the studies were free from bias. Results from the CVA studies were analysed using the Grading of Recommendations Assessment, Development and Evaluation (GRADE) approach and the certainty of the evidence was 'low' to 'very low'.

Safety

Chinese herbal medicine appeared to be safe for patients with chronic cough, when taken alone or when combined with other pharmacotherapies. The number of adverse events was generally less in the CHM groups and overall mild in nature and self-resolving.

Chinese Herbal Medicine Formulas

Chinese herbal medicines commonly used for chronic cough are consistent between classical literature, contemporary clinical guidelines and clinical trials (Table 8.1). Six formulas were specified in Chapter 2 based on CM syndrome differentiation: *Su huang zhi ke fang* 苏黄止咳方, *Er chen tang* 二陈汤 combined with *San zi yang qin tang* 三子养亲汤, *Qing yan li qiao tang* 清咽利窍汤, *Xuan fu dai zhe tang* 旋覆代赭汤 combined with *Ban xia xie xin tang* 半夏泻心汤, *Dai ge san* 黛蛤散 combined with *Huang qin xie bai san* 黄芩泻白散, and *Sha shen mai dong tang* 沙参麦冬汤.

A few formulas found in contemporary literature and classical literature have yet to be investigated in clinical studies for chronic cough. These formulas include *E jiao san* 阿胶散, *Bei mu tang* 贝母汤, *Bu fei tang* 补肺汤, *Ga jie wan* 蛤蚧丸, *Zi wan san* 紫菀散, *Bei mu wan* 贝母丸, *He zi yin* 诃子饮, *Jin su wan* 金粟丸, *Jiu sou wan zi* 久嗽丸子, *Ren shen kuan hua gao* 人参款花膏, *Zhi ke tang* 枳壳汤 and *Zhou fei wan* 皱肺丸. The use of these formulas is likely based on clinical experience of CM practitioners rather than on the pathogenesis of chronic cough.

Acupuncture and Related Therapies

This section summarises the evidence from Chapter 2, Chapter 3 and Chapter 7. The clinical guidelines (Chapter 2) recommend manual acupuncture on a few main acupuncture points based on syndrome differentiation. Few citations in the classical literature reported acupuncture and moxibustion for chronic cough (Chapter 3). Out of the five acupuncture clinical studies, all studies evaluated the effect of acupuncture, ear acupressure or acupuncture combined with herbal medicine on CVA. There were no CCTs or non-controlled clinical studies. The acupuncture therapies recommended in Chapter 2, and found in Chapter 3, have also been studied in multiple RCTs and are listed in Table 8.2. Chinese medicine syndrome differentiation was not included in the studies.

Acupuncture points described in the classical literature, contemporary guidelines and textbooks, and in clinical trials include the following:

- BL13 *Feishu* 肺俞;
- ST36 *Zusanli* 足三里;
- BL43 *Gaohuanshu* 膏肓俞;
- BL12 *Fengmen* 风门.

The points LU1 *Zhongfu* 中府, LU9 *Taiyuan* 太渊, PC6 *Neiguan* 内关, LR2 *Xingjian* 行间 and KI3 *Taixi* 太溪 were only mentioned in clinical guidelines. The points LU7 *Lieque* 列缺, ST40 *Fenglong* 丰隆, LU10 *Yuji* 鱼际 and GV14 *Dazhui* 大椎 are recommended in the clinical practice guidelines but were not mentioned in clinical trials.

Some frequently used points in clinical trials also included BL20 *Pishu* 脾俞, BL23 *Shenshu* 肾俞, EX-B1 *Dingchuan* 定喘, LU5

Table 8.2. Summary of Acupuncture and Related Therapies

Intervention	Included in Clinical Guidelines and Textbooks (Chapter 2)	Included in Classical Literature (Chapter 3) (No. of Citations)	Included in Clinical Studies (Chapter 7)			Combination Therapy with Chinese Herbal Medicine
			RCTs (No. of Studies)	CCTs (No. of Studies)	NCS (No. of Studies)	
Acupuncture	Yes	8	3	NA	NA	1
Moxibustion	Yes	19	0	NA	NA	0
Ear acupressure	No	0	1	NA	NA	0
Acupuncture and moxibustion	No	2	0	NA	NA	0
Acupuncture Points						
BL13 Feishu 肺俞	Yes	9	3	NA	NA	0
LU1 Zhongfu 中府	Yes	0	0	NA	NA	0
LU7 Lieque 列缺	Yes	0	2	NA	NA	0
LU9 Taiyuan 太渊	Yes	0	0	NA	NA	0
ST36 Zusanli 足三里	Yes	2	2	NA	NA	0
PC6 Neiguan 内关	Yes	0	0	NA	NA	0
ST40 Fenglong 丰隆	Yes	0	2	NA	NA	0
LR2 Xingjian 行间	Yes	0	0	NA	NA	0

(Continued)

Table 8.2. (*Continued*)

Intervention	Included in Clinical Guidelines and Textbooks (Chapter 2)	Included in Classical Literature (Chapter 3) (No. of Citations)	Included in Clinical Studies (Chapter 7)			Combination Therapy with Chinese Herbal Medicine
			RCTs (No. of Studies)	CCTs (No. of Studies)	NCS (No. of Studies)	
LU10 Yuji 鱼际	Yes	0	1	NA	NA	0
BL43 Gaohuanshu 膏肓俞	Yes	4	1	NA	NA	0
KI3 Taixi 太溪	Yes	0	0	NA	NA	0
GV14 Dazhui 大椎	Yes	0	1	NA	NA	0
BL12 Fengmen 风门	Yes	2	1	NA	NA	0
EX-HN10 Juquan 聚泉	No	6	0	NA	NA	0
GV10 Lingtai 灵台	No	3	0	NA	NA	0
ST18 Rugen 乳根	No	3	0	NA	NA	0
CV10 Xiawan 下脘	No	2	0	NA	NA	0
CV17 Danzhong 膻中	No	2	0	NA	NA	0
CV4 Guanyuan 关元	No	2	0	NA	NA	0
ST12 Quepen 缺盆	No	2	0	NA	NA	0
TE10 Tianjing 天井	No	2	0	NA	NA	0
BL20 Pishu 脾俞	No	0	2	NA	NA	0

The total number of studies in each section included 29 classical literature citations, five RCTs, 0 CCTs and 0 non-controlled studies.
Abbreviations: CCTs, controlled clinical trials; NA, not applicable; NCS, non-controlled studies; RCTs, randomised controlled trials.

Chize 尺泽, and ear points CO14 *Lung* 肺, TF4 *Shenmen* 神门, TG3 *Throat* 咽喉, CO16 *Trachea* 气管 and *Asthma* 平喘点. The points EX-HN10 *Juquan* 聚泉, GV10 *Lingtai* 灵台, ST18 *Rugen* 乳根, CV10 *Xiawan* 下脘, CV17 *Danzhong* 膻中, CV4 *Guanyuan* 关元, ST12 *Quepen* 缺盆 and TE10 *Tianjing* 天井 were identified in the classical literature but not mentioned in clinical practice guidelines or clinical trials.

Evidence from acupuncture RCTs showed a trend towards improvement in cough symptoms, lung function and eosinophil counts. However, the studies had small sample sizes, and a clear understanding of acupuncture's effect on chronic cough cannot be drawn from these studies, yet the results are encouraging.

Safety

One acupuncture study reported adverse events in both groups. However, the severity of adverse events was not reported in either group. Combination therapy studies of CHM and acupuncture showed acupuncture plus CHM can improve FEV_1 and reduce eosinophils, compared to montelukast. However, there were methodological shortfalls and it is difficult to draw a reliable conclusion on the efficacy and safety of combination therapies for chronic cough.

Limitations of Evidence

Significant effort was made to collect and analyse data from a range of sources, yet omissions from each of the datasets are possible. The overview of current CM clinical practice in Chapter 2 is taken from authoritative clinical practice guidelines and textbooks. However, this is not a comprehensive list and some syndromes and treatments which are not widely used are not included in Chapter 2. In addition, recommendations may change in the future.

The classical literature in Chapter 3 is a comprehensive summary of the treatment of chronic cough in pre-modern China. Three search terms were used to find the chronic cough citations, yet searching more terms may have found more citations. In terms of the search results, the evidence of acupuncture and related therapies for chronic cough was limited and it is unknown if acupuncture was historically used for this condition.

Clinical trial evidence presented in Chapters 5 and 7 includes literature from a comprehensive search of the Chinese and English scientific databases. However, errors or misclassification may have occurred during the screening process. When appropriate, meta-analysis was conducted to provide aggregate data from multiple studies. The evidence for CM interventions, compared to placebo or conventional treatments such as ICS plus bronchodilator, showed consistent results in favour of CHM/acupuncture or integrative medicine (CHM/acupuncture plus ICS and bronchodilator). Of studies included in meta-analysis, variations such as demographic features, co-morbidity and outcome measurements were considerable. Consequently, substantial statistical heterogeneity was observed in pooled results that could not be explained by subgroup analysis. To account for the heterogeneity, a random effects model was used to provide conservative estimations of effect sizes. In addition, methodological quality of most studies is 'moderate' to 'very low'. Limitations include insufficient random allocation procedures, lack of blinding of participants and personnel, and small sample sizes.

Studies evaluating acupuncture were few in number and a firm conclusion could not be drawn from the current clinical evidence. Compared with pharmacotherapy, acupuncture plus pharmacotherapy was superior in terms of effective rate, FEV_1, FVC and PEF. Compared with pharmacotherapy, ear acupressure plus pharmacotherapy was superior in terms of cough symptom score. However, there were only a small number of studies with small sample sizes and the true effect remains unclear. No clinical evidence of other CM therapies was available for synthesis. More clinical trials are needed to evaluate the effect of other CM therapies.

CHM and acupuncture given together was assessed in only one clinical trial. Compared with pharmacotherapy, acupuncture combined with herbal medicine was superior in terms of FEV_1, FVC, PEF and eosinophils. Therefore, it was difficult to draw a firm conclusion on their efficacy for chronic cough. The limitations discussed above should be taken into consideration when interpreting the results in this book.

Implications for Practice

A summary of information from the clinical guidelines and textbooks (Chapter 2) provides important guidance for syndrome differentiation and selection of appropriate CM treatments for people with chronic cough. Chronic cough, which lasts for more than eight weeks, is associated with significant morbidity and impairs quality of life. The three most common types of chronic cough, accounting for approximately 90% of cases, include CVA, UACS and GORD-C. The main organs involved, in terms of CM theory, are the Lung, Liver, Spleen, Stomach and Kidney. Severe wind attacking the Lungs has been described across clinical guidelines and clinical trial evidence, and should be considered the main syndrome for chronic cough.

Chinese herbal medicine or acupuncture alone, or combined with pharmacotherapy, improve health-related quality of life and lung function. The most commonly studied herbs with a favourable effect for chronic cough are *gan cao* 甘草 (including *zhi gan cao* 炙甘草), *chan tui* 蝉蜕, *jie geng* 桔梗, *xing ren* 杏仁 and *wu wei zi* 五味子. The evidence of acupuncture on chronic cough is limited, but results from clinical trials are promising. The most commonly studied acupuncture points with favourable effects are BL13, LU7, ST36 and ST40. Taken together, these findings indicate CHM and acupuncture may improve health-related quality of life and lung function and could be considered as part of an overall treatment plan for people with chronic cough.

Implications for Research

Many clinical studies evaluated the efficacy and safety of CM therapies for chronic cough. Encouraging evidence is available for CHM and acupuncture therapies, but evidence is lacking for other therapies. Further clinical research will increase knowledge and help to improve the management of chronic cough. Despite the common use of several herbs in clinical studies, pre-clinical studies relevant to chronic cough were limited. Future experimental studies will also improve the understanding of their mechanisms of action and may lead to new therapeutic agents.

Clinical Trial Design

Rigorous methodology is needed when designing future clinical trials of CM therapies for chronic cough. Methods of sequence generation and allocation concealment should be clearly stated. Due to the nature of acupuncture practice, blinding of personnel is difficult in acupuncture studies. Future RCTs should also publish their protocols and be registered with a clinical trials registry to minimise reporting bias and increase transparency in reporting of the results.

Cause of disease and disease course should be taken into consideration when designing trials; more comparable and reliable results will be produced if similar participants are recruited. A considerable number of clinically important outcomes were reported as main outcome measures, such as effective rate, lung function, FEV_1, PEF, FVC, EOS and cough symptom score. But other cough severity instruments were not commonly used, such as the LCQ, VAS, ECP, FeNO and cough reflex sensitivity. Assessing these outcomes may provide a better understanding of the effect of CM therapies for chronic cough.

The majority of clinical trials included treatment for five days to 14 weeks, and only a few reported follow-up data. Chronic cough is a protracted disease and follow-up assessments would provide long-term evidence of CM therapies for chronic cough and further strengthen the evidence. In addition, most studies did not specify the use of CM syndromes for selection of CHM. Where possible, CM treatments should be based on syndrome differentiation. This will help to improve translation of results into clinical practice.

The majority of RCTs included in this book were assessed as 'unclear' risk of bias for many domains due to insufficiency of details provided. Future clinical studies should follow the items required by the Consolidated Standards of Reporting Trials (CONSORT)[4] and its extensions for herbal medicine, traditional CM and acupuncture.[5–8] Informative reporting of trial participants, reasons for intervention selection, comparator and results of validated outcome measures will provide high-level clinical evidence and benefit practitioners, researchers and patients.

References

1. Gibson PG, Vertigan AE. (2015) Management of chronic refractory cough. *BMJ* **14 351:** h5590.
2. Irwin RS, French CL, Chang AB, Altman KW. (2018) Classification of cough as a symptom in adults and management algorithms: CHEST Guideline and Expert Panel Report. *Chest* **153(1):** 196–209.
3. Kahrilas PJ, Altman KW, Chang AB, *et al.* (2016) Chronic cough due to gastroesophageal reflux in adults: CHEST Guideline and Expert Panel Report. *Chest* **150(6):** 1341–1360.
4. Schulz KF, Altman DG, Moher D. (2010) CONSORT 2010 statement: Updated guidelines for reporting parallel group randomised trials. *BMJ* **340:** c332.
5. Gagnier JJ, Boon H, Rochon P, *et al.* (2006). Reporting randomized, controlled trials of herbal interventions: An elaborated CONSORT statement. *Ann Intern Med* **144(5):** 364–367.
6. Bian Z, Liu B, Moher D, *et al.* (2011) Consolidated standards of reporting trials (CONSORT) for traditional Chinese medicine: Current situation and future development. *Front Med* **5(2):** 171–177.
7. MacPherson H, White A, Cummings M, *et al.* (2002) Standards for reporting interventions in controlled trials of acupuncture: The STRICTA recommendations. Standards for Reporting Interventions in Controlled Trials of Acupuncture. *Acupunct Med* **20(1):** 22–25.
8. MacPherson H, Altman DG, Hammerschlag R, *et al.* (2010) Revised Standards for Reporting Interventions in Clinical Trials of Acupuncture (STRICTA): Extending the CONSORT statement. *J Evid Based Med* **3(3):** 140–155.

Glossary

Terms	Acronym	Definition	Reference
95% confidence interval	95% CI	A measure of the uncertainty around the main finding of a statistical analysis. Estimates of unknown quantities, such as the odds ratio comparing an experimental intervention with a control, are usually presented as a point estimate and a 95% confidence interval. This means that if someone were to keep repeating a study in other samples from the same population, 95% of the confidence intervals from those studies would contain the true value of the unknown quantity. Alternatives to 95%, such as 90% and 99% confidence intervals, are sometimes used. Wider intervals indicate lower precision; narrow intervals, greater precision.	https://training.cochrane.org/handbook
Acupressure	—	Application of pressure on acupuncture points.	—
Acupuncture	—	The insertion of needles into humans or animals for remedial purposes.	World Health Organisation. (2007) WHO International Standard Terminologies of Traditional Medicine in the Western Pacific Region.
Allied and Complementary Medicine Database	AMED	Alternative medicine bibliographic database.	https://www.ebsco.com/products/research-databases/allied-and-complementary-medicine-database-amed

(*Continued*)

(Continued)

Terms	Acronym	Definition	Reference
Angiotensin-converting enzyme inhibitors	ACE inhibitors	A protease inhibitor found in serum that promotes vasodilation by blocking the formation of angiotensin II and slowing the degradation of bradykinin and other kinins. Angiotensin-converting enzyme inhibitors decrease sodium retention, water retention, blood pressure and heart size, and increase cardiac output.	Harris P, Nagy S, Vardaxis N. (2019) *Mosby's Dictionary of Medicine, Nursing and Health Professions.* Elsevier, Australia.
Australian New Zealand Clinical Trial Registry	ANZCTR	Clinical trial registry based in Australia.	www.anzctr.org.au/
Bronchoconstriction		A narrowing of the lumen of the bronchi, restricting airflow to and from the lungs.	Harris P, Nagy S, Vardaxis N. (2019) *Mosby's Dictionary of Medicine, Nursing and Health Professions.* Elsevier, Australia.
China National Knowledge Infrastructure	CNKI	Chinese language bibliographic database.	www.cnki.net
Chinese Biomedical Literature Database	CBM	Chinese language bibliographic database.	www.imicams.ac.cn
Chinese Clinical Trial Registry	ChiCTR	Chinese clinical trial registry.	http://www.chictr.org.cn/
Chinese herbal medicine	CHM	Chinese herbal medicine.	—
Chinese medicine	CM	—	—
Chongqing VIP Information Company	CQVIP	Chinese language bibliographic database.	www.cqvip.com
ClinicalTrials.gov	—	Clinical trial registry based in the United States.	https://clinicaltrials.gov/
Cochrane Central Register of Controlled Trials	CENTRAL	Bibliographic database that provides a highly concentrated source of reports of controlled trials.	https://community.cochrane.org/editorial-and-publishing-policy-resource/ overview-cochrane-library-and-related-

(Continued)

Terms	Acronym	Definition	Reference
			content/databases-included-cochrane-library/cochrane-central-register-controlled-trials-central
Combination therapies	—	Two or more Chinese medicines from different therapy groups (e.g. Chinese herbal medicine, acupuncture therapies or other Chinese medicine therapies) administered together.	—
Controlled clinical trials	CCT	A study in which people are allocated to different interventions using methods that are not random.	https://training.cochrane.org/handbook
Convention on International Trade in Endangered Species of Wild Fauna and Flora	CITES	International convention aimed at preventing or regulating trade in threatened and endangered species of plants and animals.	https://www.cites.org/eng/disc/text.php
Cough variant asthma	CVA	Asthma characterised by minimal wheezing and a non-productive cough.	Harris P, Nagy S, Vardaxis N. (2019) *Mosby's Dictionary of Medicine, Nursing and Health Professions.* Elsevier, Australia.
Cumulative Index of Nursing and Allied Health Literature	CINAHL	Bibliographic database.	https://www.ebscohost.com/nursing/products/cinahl-databases
Effect size	—	A generic term for the estimate of the effect of a treatment in a study.	http://handbook.cochrane.org/
Effective rate	—	A measure of the proportion of participants who achieved an improvement, as outlined in Chapter 4.	—
European Clinical Trials Register	EU-CTR	European clinical trial registry.	https://www.clinicaltrialsregister.eu
Excerpta Medica database	Embase	Bibliographic database.	http://www.elsevier.com/solutions/embase

(Continued)

(*Continued*)

Terms	Acronym	Definition	Reference
Gastro-oesophageal reflux disease-related cough	GORD-C	Cough related to a backflow of contents from the stomach into the oesophagus that is often the result of incompetence of the lower oesophageal sphincter.	Harris P, Nagy S, Vardaxis N. (2019) *Mosby's Dictionary of Medicine, Nursing and Health Professions.* Elsevier, Australia.
Grading of Recommendations Assessment, Development, and Evaluation	GRADE	Approach used to grade quality of evidence and strength of recommendations.	http://www.gradeworkinggroup.org/
Heterogeneity	—	Used in a general sense to describe the variation in, or diversity of, participants, interventions and measurement of outcomes across a set of studies, or the variation in internal validity of those studies. Used specifically, as statistical heterogeneity, to describe the degree of variation in the effect estimates from a set of studies. Also used to indicate the presence of variability among studies beyond the amount expected due solely to the play of chance.	https://training.cochrane.org/handbook
Homogeneity	—	Used in a general sense to mean that the participants, interventions and measurement of outcomes are similar across a set of studies. Used specifically to describe the effect estimates from a set of studies where they do not vary more than would be expected by chance.	https://training.cochrane.org/handbook
I^2	—	A measure of study heterogeneity; indicates the percentage of variance in a meta-analysis.	https://training.cochrane.org/handbook
Integrative medicine	—	The integration of holistic and complementary medicine with current mainstream medical practice. In this book it refers to Chinese medicine treatments combined with pharmacotherapy or other conventional therapy.	Harris P, Nagy S, Vardaxis N. (2019) *Mosby's Dictionary of Medicine, Nursing and Health Professions.* Elsevier, Australia.

(Continued)

Terms	Acronym	Definition	Reference
Mean difference	MD	In meta-analysis, a method used to combine measures on continuous scales, where the mean, standard deviation and sample size in each group are known. The weight given to the difference in means from each study (e.g. how much influence each study has on the overall results of the meta-analysis) is determined by the precision of its estimate of effect; mathematically this is equal to the inverse of the variance. This method assumes that all of the trials have measured the outcome on the same scale.	https://training.cochrane.org/handbook
Meta-analysis	—	A qualitive method of evaluating statistical data based on results of several independent studies of the same topic. The results are summarised as one large study.	Harris P, Nagy S, Vardaxis N. (2019) *Mosby's Dictionary of Medicine, Nursing and Health Professions*. Elsevier, Australia.
Moxibustion	—	A therapeutic procedure involving ignited material (usually moxa) to apply heat to certain points or areas of the body surface for managing disease.	World Health Organisation. (2007) WHO International Standard Terminologies of Traditional Medicine in the Western Pacific Region.
Non-controlled studies	—	Observations made on individuals, usually receiving the same intervention, before and after the intervention but with no control group.	https://training.cochrane.org/handbook
Other Chinese medicine therapies	—	Other Chinese medicine therapies include all traditional therapies except Chinese herbal medicine and acupuncture/moxibustion, such as *tai chi* 太极, *qigong* 气功, *tuina* 推拿 and cupping.	
PubMed	PubMed	Bibliographic database.	http://www.ncbi.nlm.nih.gov/pubmed

(Continued)

(*Continued*)

Terms	Acronym	Definition	Reference
Randomised controlled trial	RCT	Clinical trial that uses a random method to allocate participants to treatment and control groups.	—
Reflux	—	An abnormal backward or return flow of a fluid.	Harris P, Nagy S, Vardaxis N. (2019) *Mosby's Dictionary of Medicine, Nursing and Health Professions*. Elsevier, Australia.
Risk of bias	—	Assessment of clinical trials to indicate if the results may overestimate or underestimate the true effect because of bias in study design or reporting.	https://training.cochrane. org/handbook
Risk ratio (relative risk)	RR	The ratio of risks in two groups. In intervention studies, it is the ratio of the risk in the intervention group to the risk in the control group. A risk ratio of 1 indicates no difference between comparison groups. For undesirable outcomes, a risk ratio that is less than 1 indicates that the intervention was effective in reducing the risk of that outcome.	https://training.cochrane. org/handbook
Standardised mean difference	SMD	In meta-analysis, a method used to combine results for continuous scales which measure the same outcome, but measure it in different ways (e.g. with different scales). The results of studies are standardised to a uniform scale to allow data to be combined.	https://training.cochrane. org/handbook
Summary of findings	SoF	Presentation of results and rating the quality of evidence based on the GRADE approach.	http://www. gradeworkinggroup.org/
Upper airway cough syndrome	UACS	A syndrome characterised by chronic cough related to upper airway abnormalities. Upper airway cough syndrome commonly involves a sensation of something draining into the	Pratter M. (2006) Chronic upper airway cough syndrome secondary to rhinosinus diseases (previously referred to as postnasal drip

Terms	Acronym	Definition	Reference
		throat, a need to clear the throat, a tickle in the throat, nasal congestion or a nasal discharge.	syndrome): ACCP evidence-based clinical practice guidelines. *Chest* **129(Suppl 1):** S63–S71.
Wanfang database	Wanfang	Chinese language bibliographic database.	www.wanfangdata.com
World Health Organisation	WHO	World Health Organisation is the directing and coordinating authority for health within the United Nations system. It is responsible for providing leadership on global health matters, shaping the health research agenda, setting norms and standards, articulating evidence-based policy options, providing technical support to countries, and monitoring and assessing health trends.	http://www.who.int/about/en/
Zhong Hua Yi Dian 中华医典	ZHYD	The *Zhong Hua Yi Dian* [Encyclopaedia of Traditional Chinese Medicine] is a comprehensive series of electronic books on compact disk. The collection was put together by the Hunan Electronic and Audio-visual Publishing House. It is the largest collection of Chinese electronic books and includes the major Chinese ancient works, many of which are from rare manuscripts and are the only existing copies. These books cover the period from ancient times up to the period of the Republic of China (1911–1948).	Hu R, ed. (2014) *Zhong Hua Yi Dian* [*Encyclopaedia of Traditional Chinese Medicine*], 5th ed Hunan Electronic and Audio-Visual Publishing House, Chengsha.
Zhong Yi Fang Ji Da Ci Dian 中医方剂大辞典	ZYFJDCD	Compendium of Chinese herbal formulas with over 96,592 entries derived from classical Chinese books. The Nanjing Chinese Medicine Institute compiled the *Zhong Yi Fang Ji Da Ci Dian* and first published it in 1993.	Peng HR, ed. (1994) *Zhong Yi Fang Ji Da Ci Dian* [*Great Compendium of Chinese Medical Formulae*]. People's Medical Publishing House, Beijing.

Index

gastro-oesophageal reflux disease-
related cough, 3, 135–137, 139
GORD, 9–11, 51
GORD-C, 3, 12
GRADE, 111–116, 119–121

H
heat, 34, 48, 193

J
jie geng, 23, 133, 165–167
jiu ke, 18, 29, 31, 33
jiu sou, 18, 29, 31, 32

K
Kidney, 19, 36, 203

L
Liver, 19, 24, 36, 203
low risk of bias, 55–57, 72, 73, 133
LU7 *Lieque*, 184, 189
lung function, 79, 86, 89, 130, 187
Lungs, 17–24, 34

M
ma huang, 159–161, 163
moxibustion, 27, 45, 46, 48, 49

N
non-controlled studies, 51–53

O
other CM therapies, 32, 33, 47, 49
outcomes, 54, 55, 57–59

P
peak expiratory flow (PEF), 70,
187, 196
phlegm, 17, 19–26
phlegm-dampness, 19, 22, 66

placebo, 72, 77, 103, 196, 202
proton pump inhibitors, 192

Q
qi, 23, 34–36, 192, 193

R
randomised controlled trials
(RCTs), 51, 62, 157
reflux, 3, 7–10, 12, 135–137, 139,
158
regurgitation, 3, 12, 23, 192
risk of bias, 55–58, 68, 69, 186,
196

S
severe wind attacking the Lungs,
19–21, 203
Spleen, 19, 35
ST36 *Zusanli*, 26, 184, 189
ST40 *Fenglong*, 26, 184, 186, 189
Stomach, 18–20, 23–26
Su huang zhi ke fang, 66, 74, 76,
85, 94, 98
syndrome classification, 102, 107,
132
systematic reviews, 62, 183

T
Tan yin ke sou, 31, 32, 33

U
UACS, 11–13, 51, 53, 57
upper airway cough syndrome, 1,
3, 6, 9, 64, 140

V
visual analogue scale, 70, 77–79,
138

W

wan ke, 18
Wen dan tang, 66, 67, 123, 136
wu wei zi, 160, 168, 169

X

Xiao qing long tang, 66, 107, 110,
  122, 131
xing ren, 43, 160, 163, 164

Z

Zhi sou san, 66, 86, 94, 107, 110,
  122
zi su ye, 160, 171, 172
zi wan, 160, 169, 170

Forthcoming

9 789811 235436